MANAGING LONG-TERM CONDITIONS AND CHRONIC ILLNESS IN PRIMARY CARE

Effective management of long-term conditions is an important aspect of contemporary nursing policy and practice. Systematic and evidence-based care which takes account of the expert patient and reduces unnecessary hospital admissions is vital to support those with long-term conditions/chronic illnesses and those who care for them.

This book draws together the key issues in managing long-term conditions and provides a practical and accessible guide for nurses and allied health professionals in the primary care environment. It covers background context and policy in the UK and further afield, as well as practical guidance for all key aspects of long-term condition management, including:

- the physical and psychosocial impact of long-term conditions;
- effective case management;
- self-management and the expert patient;
- behavioural change strategies and motivational counselling;
- nutritional and medication management.

Packed with helpful, clearly written information, *Managing Long-term Conditions and Chronic Illness in Primary Care* includes a chapter of case scenarios as well as key fact boxes and pointers for practice throughout. It is suitable for pre-registration students undertaking community placements and post-registration students studying long-term condition/chronic illness management.

Judith Carrier is Lecturer and Professional Head of Primary Care/Public Health Nursing at Cardiff University, UK, where she is responsible for practice nurse education. She has a regular column in *Practice Nursing*.

MANAGING LONG-TERM CONDITIONS AND CHRONIC ILLNESS IN PRIMARY CARE

A guide to good practice

Judith Carrier

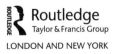

Routledge
Taylor & Francis Group

LONDON AND NEW YORK

First published 2009
by Routledge
2 Park Square, Milton Park, Abingdon, Oxon OX14 4RN

Simultaneously published in the USA and Canada
by Routledge
270 Madison Avenue, New York, NY 10016

Reprinted 2009, 2010

Routledge is an imprint of the Taylor & Francis Group, an informa business

Typeset in Sabon and Futura by
Keystroke, 28 High Street, Tettenhall, Wolverhampton
Printed and bound in Great Britain by
TJ International Ltd, Padstow, Cornwall

British Library Cataloguing in Publication Data
A catalogue record for this book is available from the British Library

Library of Congress Cataloging in Publication Data
Carrier, Judith, 1960–
Managing long-term conditions and chronic illness in primary care:
a guide to good practice/Judith Carrier.
p. cm.
1. Chronic diseases–Nursing. 2. Primary care (Medicine) I. Title.
[DNLM: 1. Chronic Disease–nursing. 2. Nursing Care–methods.
3. Case Management. 4. Primary Health Care. WY 152 C316m 2009]
RC108.C37 2009
610.73–dc22   2008038202

ISBN 10: 0–415–45087–X (hbk)
ISBN 10: 0–415–45088–8 (pbk)
ISBN 10: 0–203–88131–1 (ebk)

ISBN 13: 978–0–415–45087–4 (hbk)
ISBN 13: 978–0–415–45088–1 (pbk)
ISBN 13: 978–0–203–88131–6 (ebk)

This book is dedicated to my father Reginald Henson who lost his battle against chronic illness on 4 January 2000 and to my mother Barbara Henson who battles on and lives life to the full despite chronic back pain, osteoporosis and osteoarthritis.

The author's royalties from this book will be donated to the following charities:

- Friends of Bwindi, which supports orphaned and vulnerable children living in the village of Bwindi in the Bwindi Impenetrable Rainforest, South Western Uganda, home to half of the world's mountain gorillas;
- and The Gorilla Organization, an international charity led by experienced African conservationists, dedicated to saving the world's last remaining gorillas from extinction.

Thanks

CONTENTS

ILLUSTRATIONS

FIGURES

TABLES

CONTRIBUTORS

Rhiannon Britton graduated as a state registered dietitian from the University Wales Institute, Cardiff (UWIC) in 2007, with a BSc (Hons) in Dietetics and Nutrition. She is currently working for the NHS with a focus on patients recovering from stroke. She has a keen interest in health and nutrition and the role of food in chronic disease/long-term condition management.

Claire A. Lane is originally from a linguistics background, and undertook her PhD in healthcare communication in the Department of General Practice, Cardiff University. Her academic work to date has focused on Motivational Interviewing (MI), and more specifically the teaching of MI to practitioners working in a wide range of healthcare contexts. To this end, her PhD study examined effects of training on practitioner skill in motivational interviewing, and involved the development of an instrument to measure this (The Behaviour Change Counselling Index, or 'BECCI'). Claire is currently working in the Cardiff University School of Nursing and Midwifery Studies, investigating the transition of patients from paediatric to adult diabetes services.

Gina Newbury is a lecturer and programme manager for the BSc Community Health Studies programme at Cardiff University School of Nursing and Midwifery Studies. She completed both her general and district nurse training in Cardiff, working as a district nurse team leader before moving into education. Her dissertation for her recently completed Masters in Education focused on the future development of community nursing education.

Meryl Prosser completed her general nurse training at St Mary's Hospital, London before taking a degree in Social History and Social Policy at Swansea University. She then trained as a health visitor at Bulmershe College, Reading and practiced health visiting for several years before becoming a lecturer at Cardiff University School of Nursing and Midwifery Studies, where her interests are mainly in Health Promotion and Social Policy.

ACKNOWLEDGEMENTS

I would like to thank the following friends and colleagues for their help and support in putting this book together:

- Dr Claire Lane for sharing her expertise and providing the chapter on motivational interviewing;
- Meryl Prosser, my office buddy and constant source of support and encouragement, for the section in Chapter 2 on social influences on health;
- Gina Newbury, my close friend and colleague, for her contribution on the district nursing role in Chapter 3;
- Rhiannon Britton for writing the section on dietary management in Chapter 10 and reminding me of the importance of including it in this book!
- Cathy Stracey, respiratory specialist nurse, for supplying ideas for the asthma/COPD case studies;
- Dr Julian Costello for his advice on read codes;
- Professor Paul Bennett for proofreading the section on psychological impact;
- Sally Rees for lending me all her articles on self-management and proof-reading Chapter 4;
- Angela Bowyer, librarian, for helping to locate relevant documents and studies.

Thanks to the following organisations for allowing me permission to reproduce work previously published by them:

- *Practice Nursing*
- NHS Institute for Innovation and Improvement.

Finally, last but not least, thanks to my family: John for buying me a new computer, fixing it when it went wrong and not moaning too much about the time I spent on it, and my son and daughter Ben and Sam, just for being there.

CHAPTER 1

SOCIAL AND POLITICAL BACKGROUND

OVERVIEW

This chapter sets the scene, beginning with a definition of chronic disease/long-term condition (LTC) management. It provides an overview of the current incidence and prevalence of LTCs in the UK and further afield. The current UK policy drivers leading the way forward are discussed including National Service Frameworks (NSFs), National Institute of Clinical Excellence (NICE) guidelines and the Quality and Outcomes Framework (QOF) in the new General Medical Services (nGMS) contract. Theoretical frameworks and service delivery models, which were initiated in the USA and have been adapted both in the UK and other countries, such as the Chronic Care Model, Evercare and Kaiser Permanente, are introduced and discussed.

INTRODUCTION

> Chronic Diseases are diseases, which current medical interventions can only control, not cure. The life of a person with a chronic condition is forever altered – there is no return to 'normal'.
>
> (DoH 2004a, p. 3)

This statement introduces a document produced by the Department of Health (DoH), United Kingdom, in which the increasing problem of chronic disease to individuals, carers, the health service and society as a whole is emphasised, the document stating that 'the fact that chronic disease is the biggest problem facing health care services worldwide seems unarguable' (DoH 2004a, p.3). Wilson *et al.* (2005) note that the new challenge to health care systems, of supporting people with LTCs, is a direct result of the health gains of the past 50 years, improvements in public health leading to an increased ageing population, who are less susceptible to events such as serious infections that previously proved fatal, but are increasingly likely to develop a long-term condition. A joint publication from the Welsh Assembly Government (WAG) and the National Public Health Service – Wales (NPHS) (2005) notes that patterns of disease are subject to continual change and that the current burden of disease is shifting both from the young to the old and from communicable to non-communicable (chronic) diseases. The DoH (2004b) outlines the problem associated with LTCs in the National Health Service (NHS) improvement plan, stating that:

> As people live longer, growing numbers of people have medical conditions that they will live with for the rest of their lives. These long-term illnesses are increasingly common and the ability to respond well to the needs of patients with them has become an important part of modern healthcare.

This increasing health care problem is not one restricted to the UK, or even Europe; many countries, including the USA, Canada, Australia and New Zealand and some Asian countries, are increasingly directing their health care strategies towards tackling the challenges presented by the problem of chronic disease, both physical and mental. Indeed, the World Health Organisation (WHO) produced a global report in 2002, *Innovative Care for Chronic Conditions*, in which it notes:

> Chronic conditions share fundamental themes: they persist and they require some level of health care management across time. In addition, chronic conditions share some concerning features:
>
> - Chronic conditions are increasing throughout the world, and no country is immune to their impact.
> - Chronic conditions seriously challenge the efficiency and effectiveness of current health care systems and test our abilities to organize systems to meet the imminent demands.
> - Chronic conditions engender increasingly serious economic and social consequences in all regions and threaten health care resources in every country.
> - Chronic conditions can be curtailed, but only when leaders in government and healthcare embrace change and innovation.
>
> (WHO 2002b, p. 11)

The WHO (2002b) notes that current health care systems were initially developed to respond to acute problems and urgent patient need: testing, diagnosing, relieving symptoms and expecting to cure all hallmarks of contemporary health care. It further adds that this acute care template is clearly not suitable for patients with chronic problems and an evolution in health care systems is imperative if the needs of those with chronic problems are to be met. Without doubt the impact of chronic conditions on both individuals and providers of health care is set to increase, and it is vital that all health care professionals remain aware of the challenges that this presents.

The term 'long-term condition' is now increasingly favoured as an alternative to the term 'chronic disease' or 'chronic illness', and will be the one generally used throughout this book, except when citing work where an alternative term has been used by an author or an organisation.

INCIDENCE AND PREVALENCE

More than 17.5 million adults in the UK are estimated to report a chronic health problem (DoH 2005a). Based on population surveys (self-reported as opposed to clinical data) the WAG/NPHS (2005) report *A Profile of Long Term and Chronic Conditions in Wales* noted that 23 per cent of adults in Wales reported having a long-term illness. The Scottish government publication (2007a), *Characteristics of Adults in Scotland with Long Term Conditions*, indicates that in 2005 to 2006 23.6 per cent of adults aged 16 or over reported some form of long-term illness, health problem or disability and that this prevalence has changed little since 1999. Figures for 2006 to 2007 from the QOF (DoH 2008b) indicate that 15.4 million people (33.2 per cent of the overall population) in England have a long-term condition.

The WAG/NPHS report states that although it is difficult to predict the prevalence and impact of chronic conditions in the future, based on demographic trends it is estimated that by 2014 there will be a 12 per cent increase in the number of adults with at least one chronic condition and a 20 per cent increase in those aged 65 and over with a chronic condition. It is also emphasised that until recently there were a limited number of data sources that could provide information on chronic conditions in Wales or comparisons across the UK, as much of the information came from population surveys which relied on self-reported rather than clinical data. This explains the difficulty in obtaining exact

Table 1.1 Definition of terms

- Incidence: Number of new cases within a given period
- Prevalence: Number of existing cases at a given period in time

prevalence rates and the consequent discrepancies related to prevalence data obtained from different sources. Data from the General Medical Services (GMS) Quality and Outcomes Framework (QOF) (BMA/NHS Confederation 2003), through which GPs supply information in relation to chronic disease prevalence and quality indicators, now allow for a more accurate picture, but at the time of writing the QOF still does not include all chronic conditions and does not distinguish between those suffering from single or multiple chronic conditions.

Prevalence of LTCs also increases with age. The DoH (2005a) estimated that up to three-quarters of people aged over 75 were suffering from chronic illness, with 45 per cent of those having more than one condition. Sixty per cent of those aged 65 and over say they have an LTC (DoH 2008b). The WAG (2006b) notes that two-thirds of people in Wales aged 65 and over reported having at least one chronic condition, with one-third of those reporting multiple chronic conditions. Over three-quarters of people aged over 85 in Wales reported having a limiting long-term illness. In Scotland 54.1 per cent of people over the age of 75 reported having an LTC in 2005/2006 (Scottish Government 2007a). With the increase in the ageing population these figures are predicted to continue to grow and the impact on the NHS is considerable, with some of these issues outlined in Table 1.2.

The WHO (2007) is leading the way with the development of a comprehensive strategy to tackle the problem. The Organisation's statistics indicate that non-communicable diseases cause 86 per cent of deaths and 77 per cent of the disease burden in the WHO European Region. The conditions making up this group include cardiovascular diseases, cancer, mental health problems, diabetes mellitus, chronic respiratory disease and musculoskeletal conditions, with cardiovascular diseases noted as the number one killer, responsible for more than half the deaths across the region.

Europe is not alone in this problem; 51.6 per cent of Australians are estimated to suffer from a long-term condition (Australian Government Department of Health and Ageing 2006). Indeed, in a National Health Survey carried out in 2001(Australian Institute of Health and Welfare (AIHW) 2005) 78 per cent of respondents said they had one or more long-term health

Table 1.2 Impact of LTCs

- People with LTCs are the most intensive users of the most expensive services.
- Numbers are increasing due to factors such as an ageing population, health inequalities and certain lifestyle choices that people make.
- People with long-term conditions are not just high users of primary and specific acute services but also social care and community services and urgent and emergency care.
- Ill health among the working population places a significant burden on health and social care.
- Long-term conditions are by far the leading cause of mortality in the world.
- There are huge benefits to the population and financial savings if health and social care communities invest in effective LTC management.

(DoH 2007)

conditions (one that has lasted or is expected to last for six months or more). The AIHW uses the term DALYs – 'disability adjusted life-years' – as a measure of the years of healthy life lost due to illness or injury. One DALY is equivalent to one lost year of health life, calculated through a combination of years of life lost due to premature mortality and years of healthy life lost due to poor health or disability. In 1996 the 12 key chronic diseases (Table 1.3) were estimated to be responsible for about 42 per cent of total DALYs, since which time the burden of chronic disease has increased considerably.

Figures from New Zealand (WHO 2002a) state that chronic diseases accounted for 92 per cent of all deaths in 2002, the biggest killer being cardio-vascular disease at 42 per cent, closely followed by cancer at 27 per cent, chronic respiratory disease at 7 per cent, diabetes at 3 per cent (although as shall be seen later, deaths associated with diabetes are often due to cardiovascular disease, with diabetes rarely attributed as the defining cause) and all other chronic diseases at 14 per cent.

Chronic diseases – such as heart disease, cancer and diabetes – are the leading causes of death and disability in the United States. Chronic diseases are responsible for 70 per cent (1.7 million people) of all deaths in the USA each year, with more than 90 million Americans living with chronic illness and one-third of the years of potential life lost before the age of 65 attributed to chronic illness (Centers for Disease Control and Prevention (CDCP) 2007). In addition to the increased mortality associated with chronic disease CDCP notes that it also has a serious impact on overall quality of life, with one in ten Americans reporting severe lifestyle limitations, with the extended pain, suffering and reduced quality of life resulting from the illness and disability of chronic disease affecting millions.

Throughout England (and it is likely that this applies to most countries where LTCs are a problem), prevalence varies across regions. No single factor correlates with this prevalence and it appears that a number of factors drive this variation, including age, socioeconomic status, lifestyle choices and rurality, age being the most significant driver (DoH 2008b).

Table 1.3 The 12 key chronic diseases

Coronary heart disease (CHD)
Stroke
Chronic obstructive pulmonary disease (COPD)
Depression
Lung cancer
Diabetes
Arthritis
Colorectal cancer
Asthma
Kidney disease
Oral diseases
Osteoporosis

(AIHW 2005)

CURRENT POLICY DRIVERS

United Kingdom

Although there is one NHS across the UK, health and social care policies vary in England, Wales, Scotland and Northern Ireland. All, however, have a similar aim, namely increasing self-care and improving the management of those with more complex LTCs, preventing hospital admissions and improving quality of life for individuals. This section will, first, discuss policy drivers that impact across the UK including NSFs, NICE guidelines and the QOF of the GMS Contract. Following this, brief descriptions of health and social care policies relevant to each of the four countries in the UK will be provided.

National Service Frameworks

NSFs are evidence-based long-term strategies for improving specific areas of care. They set measurable goals within fixed time frames. NSFs:

- set national standards and identify key interventions for a defined service or care group;
- put in place strategies to support implementation;
- establish ways to ensure progress within an agreed time scale;
- form one of a range of measures to raise quality and decrease variations in service.

(DoH 2008a)

NSFs were first introduced as part of the NHS plan consultation document (DoH 1998) and cover a wide range of topics (not all related to long-term conditions). Each of the countries in the UK, except Northern Ireland which uses a taskforce approach, has its own specific National Service Frameworks. Although they may vary slightly from country to country, what they have in common is that they all aim to detect, treat, plan and manage care for named conditions or specific groups of people from the same evidence base.

National Service Frameworks are not exclusive to the UK. Australia similarly has five supporting National Service Improvement Frameworks covering the national health priority areas of asthma; cancer; diabetes; heart, stroke and vascular disease; osteoarthritis, rheumatoid arthritis and osteoporosis. The Frameworks identify opportunities to improve prevention and care (National Health Priority Action Council (NHPAC) 2006). New Zealand is also, at the time of writing, developing a long-term conditions framework (Ministry of Health NZ 2008).

National Institute of Health and Clinical Excellence guidelines

NICE is an independent UK organisation responsible for providing national guidance on the promotion of good health and the prevention and treatment of ill-health.

NICE produces guidance in three areas of health:

- public health – guidance on the promotion of good health and the prevention of ill-health for those working in the NHS, local authorities and the wider public and voluntary sector
- health technologies – guidance on the use of new and existing medicines, treatments and procedures within the NHS
- clinical practice – guidance on the appropriate treatment and care of people with specific diseases and conditions within the NHS.

(NICE 2007)

Clinical guidelines are recommendations by NICE, based on the best available evidence, on the appropriate treatment and care of people with specific diseases and conditions within the NHS. Clinical guidelines are not intended to replace the knowledge and skills of health professionals, but are guides to assist them in their work. Good clinical guidelines can change the process of health care by improving the quality of the health care provided and subsequently improving people's chances of getting as well as possible. Clinical guidelines can:

- provide recommendations for the treatment and care of people by health professionals
- be used to develop standards to assess the clinical practice of individual health professionals
- be used in the education and training of health professionals
- help patients to make informed decisions
- improve communication between patient and health professional.

(NICE 2007)

NICE guidelines cover a wide range of topics and are by no means limited to LTCs. Topics covered relating to LTCs include diabetes, cardiovascular disease, and neurological, respiratory and musculoskeletal conditions; for a full range of topics access: http://www.nice.org.uk/guidance/index.jsp?action=by Topic.

Quality and Outcomes Framework, new General Medical Services contract

The QOF is the annual reward and incentive programme detailing general practice achievement results. QOF is a voluntary process for all surgeries across the UK and was initially introduced as part of the nGMS (BMA/NHS Confederation 2003) contract first implemented in 2004.

QOF awards practices which contract with the NHS to provide general primary care services achievement points for five domains:

- clinical – managing some of the most common chronic conditions, e.g. asthma, diabetes;
- organisational – how well the practice is organised;
- patient experience – how patients view their experience at the surgery;
- additional services – the amount of extra services offered such as child health and maternity services;
- holistic – based on points achieved across the domains (removed in later revisions).

Achievement points are awarded based on the quality of service provided relating to people with the conditions in Table 1.4; these are subject to regular revision, and at the time of publication the most recent changes had been made in 2008.

Points (and financial rewards) are given to practices relating to the achievement of specific indicators for each condition; examples of these indicators (different for each condition) are listed in Table 1.5.

The overall aim behind QOF is that through rewarding practices for providing improved quality of care linked to specific conditions overall quality of health care will be improved. However, it should be noted that not all long-term conditions, for example arthritis, are included in the list of conditions and

Table 1.4 Conditions	Table 1.5 Indicators for each condition
<ul><li>CHD</li><li>Heart failure</li><li>Stroke and trans-ischaemic attacks (TIA)</li><li>Hypertension</li><li>Diabetes mellitus</li><li>COPD</li><li>Epilepsy</li><li>Hypothyroidism</li><li>Cancer</li><li>Palliative care</li><li>Mental health</li><li>Asthma</li><li>Dementia</li><li>Depression</li><li>Chronic kidney disease (CKD)</li><li>Atrial fibrillation</li><li>Obesity</li><li>Learning disabilities</li><li>Smoking (in relation to specific LTCs)</li></ul>	<ul><li>Maintaining an accurate register of each disease area</li><li>Confirming disease diagnosis with objective measures</li><li>Recording smoking status</li><li>Smoking cessation advice</li><li>Measuring blood pressure (BP)</li><li>Achieving target BP</li><li>Cholesterol measuring</li><li>Achieving target cholesterol level</li><li>Specific reviews</li><li>Specific bloods</li><li>Flu jab</li><li>Specific therapy</li><li>Other outcomes</li></ul>

there has been concern that the care of people with conditions not listed in QOF may become neglected.

England

The DoH (2005c) published *Supporting People with Long Term Conditions. An NHS Social Care Model to Support Local Innovation and Integration*, which provided a framework 'to help local health and social care communities improve the care of people with LTCs'. The model has three key strands: infrastructure; delivery system; and better outcomes. Key to the government's current policy is involvement of service users, and results of surveys carried out are outlined in Table 1.6.

Table 1.6 Results of surveys

- Eighty-two per cent of those with an LTC say that they already play an active role in their care but they want to do more to self-care.
- More than 90 per cent are interested in being more active self-carers.
- More than 75 per cent say that if they had guidance/support from a professional or peer they would feel far more confident about taking care of their own health.
- More than 50 per cent who had seen a care professional in the past six months said they had not been encouraged to self-care.

(DoH 2005c)

The current focus of the DoH is on better LTC management, including improvements in clinical care and support in self-care. The DoH (2008b) document *Raising the Profile of Long Term Conditions Care* emphasises that people with LTCs use disproportionately both primary and secondary care services, with a small number of people accounting for a very high proportion of health care resources. They suggest a number of initiatives that can be put in place at each part of the framework to improve care. The examples they provide are as follows.

Infrastructure

Community resources service:

- Redesign to provide more services in the community.

Decision support tools and clinical information systems:

- Develop IT systems that can support information sharing.
- Remember the three Rs – registration, recall and review.
- Use the QOF to drive improvements.

- Use NSFs and NICE guidance to create a framework for decision support.

Health and social care system environment:

- local strategic partnerships;
- partnership working and collaboration.

Delivery system

Case management:

- use of risk prediction tools to stratify risk;
- a whole systems approach to support case management;
- person-centred and integrated assessment and care planning.

Disease management:

- personalised care planning and self-care support and management;
- use of specialist nurses and specialist support teams.

Supported self-care:

- self-care and self-management;
- access to self-care tools, monitoring equipment and assistive technology.

Promoting better health:

- Promote healthy lifestyles.

Better outcomes

- Empowered and informed patients;
- prepared and pro-active health and social care teams.

(DoH 2008b)

The DoH (2008b) also provides examples of a number of local achievements that have made a real difference, and it is recommended that the reader refers to this document for real-life examples of policy in action. One of the key focuses of DoH policy is the community matron programme, which will be discussed in further detail in Chapter 3. The overall national strategic direction of the DoH policy is to reduce emergency bed days and improve the level of satisfaction and support which people with LTCs are given, to enable them to be independent and in control of their condition.

Wales

In Wales the need to improve the management of chronic disease was recognised in the strategy *Designed for Life: A World Class Health Service for Wales* (WAG 2005). The policy focus for people with LTCs is summarised as follows.

Central to the delivery of chronic disease management is the primary care team, in conjunction with the voluntary sector and carers. Hospital admission will only take place when absolutely necessary, and as part of an agreed care pathway supported and understood by the relevant agencies. Specialist units within hospitals will be led by highly trained professionals. Individuals will be encouraged and helped to become 'expert patients', taking control over their care and treatment. Services will be provided as close as possible to individuals' homes (WAG 2005).

Services are currently being redesigned in Wales to develop an approach to chronic disease management that will be person-centred and include early assessment, timely diagnosis, and an appropriate level of specialist support within a multi-professional team (WAG 2006a).

At this point it is important to mention the role that the Expert Patients Programme (EPP) has taken in implementing WAG's policy of self-care. Although this programme will be discussed in further detail in Chapter 4, it is worth noting at this point that WAG has demonstrated a firm commitment to rolling out this programme over the whole of Wales by the end of 2008. As of September 2008:

- 345 EPP courses have been delivered in Wales
- 2676 people have completed an EPP course
- 130 volunteer tutors have been trained
- 17 local EPP Co-ordinators/Trainers have been employed to help support the volunteers and to manage and arrange the courses locally.

  (http://www.wales.nhs.uk/sites3/home.cfm?orgid=537)

Scotland

In Scotland the *Better Health Better Care Action Plan* (Scottish Government 2008) emphasises the need for patients with LTCs and their carers to have the information and support they need to manage their condition on a day-to-day basis. To achieve this goal the Scottish Executive is collaborating with the Long Term Conditions Alliance, which is working with people with LTCs and their carers to design services that fit the needs of the user. There is a strong focus on self-management and better communication with health and social care professionals. *Living Well with Long Term Conditions* (Scottish Government 2007b) has been published, which was produced by the Long Term Conditions

Alliance Scotland in consultation with service users and their carers to make things better for people with long-term conditions.

A National Health Information and Support service is planned, in partnership with the voluntary sector, to enable patients and carers to obtain clear, accurate information when needed.

Northern Ireland

A major initiative in Northern Ireland has been on investment in long-term conditions to use innovative new ways of bringing better care to people and reducing reliance on hospitals (Northern Ireland Executive 2008). New approaches to chronic disease management are being pursued using technology for remote monitoring of patients' vital signs in their homes to promote early intervention when problems arise and so avoid hospital admissions.

A Healthier Future: A Twenty Year Vision for Health and Well-being in Northern Ireland sets out Northern Ireland's policy (Department of Health, Social Services and Public Safety 2005) for the care of chronic conditions, of which a brief summary follows.

Chronic conditions are currently a major focus of attention for health and social services, with chronic disease managed in communities, wherever possible with support from hospital services. Patients will be referred to Chronic Condition Management (CCM) programmes run in local primary and community care facilities. Seven major service-wide CCM programmes will be established to promote chronic condition management. These will include enhanced management of: diabetes, coronary heart disease, stroke recovery, arthritis and muscular-skeletal problems, chronic obstructive pulmonary disease and asthma, depression and stress management. The programmes will be tailored for people suffering from one or more chronic condition to maximise resources. Support with self-management will enable people to take greater control of their own lives, reducing severity of symptoms and improving confidence and self-efficacy.

INTERNATIONAL MODELS OF SUPPORT FOR MANAGEMENT OF LTCS

The NHS Institute for Innovation and Improvement (2006) carried out an extensive evidence review of international, national and local thinking about different approaches to LTC management. The following summarised text is reproduced from D. Singh and C. Ham (2006) *Improving Care for People with Long-term Conditions: A Review of UK and International Frameworks*, NHS Institute for Innovation and Improvement and Health Services Management Centre, University of Birmingham, with the kind permission of the NHS Institute for Innovation and Improvement. Brief summaries of the evidence relating to evaluations of the models are included; for full evidence summaries the reader is directed to the original document, which may be accessed at: http://www.hsmc. bham.ac.uk/news/ReviewIntFrameworks-ltc.pdf.

BROAD THEORETICAL FRAMEWORKS

The Chronic Care Model

The Chronic Care Model was developed in the USA by Wagner *et al.* (2001) and has been applied in a number of developed countries. The key focus of the model is on empowering individuals with long-term conditions and linking them with supporting and pro-active teams of professionals. Central to this is acknowledging that the majority of care of chronic conditions takes place outside traditional health care settings. Six elements are seen to be centrally important to improve chronic care: *community resources, the health care system, patient self-management, decision support, delivery system redesign* and *clinical information systems.*

The key principles of the model include:

- mobilising community resources to meet the needs of people with LTCs;
- creating a culture, organisation and mechanisms that provide safe, high-quality care;
- empowering and preparing people to manage their health and health care;
- delivering effective, efficient care and self-management support;
- promoting care that is consistent with research evidence and patient preferences;
- organising patient and population data to facilitate efficient and effective care.

The model was revised in 2003 to include cultural competency, patient safety, care coordination, community policies and case management. Other countries have adapted or added to the model, including Canada, which felt it was difficult to apply to prevention and health promotion activities.

The Expanded Chronic Care Model

Based on the Chronic Care Model, this model was conceptualised by a health authority in Vancouver to include population health promotion concepts. The US Veteran Affairs Model also adds a health promotion and prevention component to elements of the model.

The NHS Institute for Innovation and Improvement (2005) provides a summary of the available evidence relating to the evaluation of the above models and concludes that although there is evidence that single or multiple components of the model can improve quality of care, clinical outcomes and health care resource use it is unclear whether all components of the model are necessary to improve chronic care.

Innovative Care for Chronic Conditions Model

Taking a different approach from the primary care perspective of the Chronic Conditions Model, the WHO (2002b) adapted it to focus on community and policy aspects of improving chronic care. The Innovative Care for Chronic Conditions Model focuses on improving care at three levels: micro level (individual and family); meso level (health care organisation and community); and macro level (policy). The NHS Institute for Innovation and Improvement (2005) notes that:

> the model suggests that positive outcomes for people with LTC's occur only when people and their families, community partners and health professionals are motivated, informed and working together. The micro level is supported by healthcare organisations and the broader community, which in turn influence and are impacted on by the broader policy environment.
>
> (http://www.hsmc.bham.ac.uk/news/
> ReviewIntFrameworks-ltc.pdf)

As in the Chronic Conditions Model, evidence was found relating to specific components of the model, but none was found that explicitly attempted to assess the evidence of the framework or the value of a policy focus (NHS Institute for Innovation and Improvement 2006).

The Public Health Model

This less well-known model was developed in the USA in the early 2000s and is similar to the Innovative Care for Chronic Conditions Model. The underlying principle of the Public Health Model is that there must be three levels of inter-vention in order to impact on the burden of chronic conditions:

- population-wide policies
- community activities
- health services (including both preventive services and ongoing care).

It is a systems-wide perspective model, including the continuum of prevention and care and emphasising the determinants of disease as well as social, cultural and economic factors that might impinge on the quality and quantity of care. The NHS Institute for Innovation and Improvement (2005) identified no studies of the implementation of the Public Health Model and no evidence of its effectiveness.

The Continuity of Care Model

Conceptualised in the 1990s, this model outlines how chronic conditions develop in response to risk factors in the community, suggesting points at which to target preventive efforts, medical intervention, treatment, rehabilitation and palliative care. At varying stages of the disease pathway the model suggests different needs for preventive interventions, treatment, rehabilitation and palliative care. No high-quality evaluation studies were identified by the NHS Institute for Innovation and Improvement (2005) regarding implementation of the model.

SERVICE DELIVERY MODELS

In addition to the broader theoretical frameworks outlined above, specific models have been developed focusing on effective service delivery to people with LTCs. Detailed below are some of the more commonly referred-to models as reviewed by the NHS Institute for Innovation and Improvement (2006).

Kaiser, Evercare and Pfizer

Approaches developed by Kaiser Permanente, Evercare (United Healthcare) and Pfizer in the USA all share a pro-active approach to managing care for people with long-term conditions. The Kaiser model focuses on integrating services and removing distinctions between primary and secondary care for people at all stages of the 'Kaiser pyramid' whereas the Evercare and Pfizer approaches focus on targeting those at highest risk of hospitalisation.

The Kaiser Permanente approach is based on the Chronic Care Model. It includes population-wide prevention as well as supported self-care, disease management and case management for highly complex patients with LTCs, stratified according to need, with intensive management targeted at those at highest risk. Kaiser focuses on integrating organisations and disciplines. All health care staff are housed together in multi-speciality centres, primary and secondary services sharing the same budget.

Evercare and Pfizer focus solely on case management. Evercare targets people at highest risk using advanced primary nurses as case managers (similar to the community matron role). The focus is on integrating social and health care to meet an individual's needs. Advanced primary nurses identify older people at high risk, assess their care needs and then coordinate their journey along a care pathway. The aim is to maintain health, detect changes and prevent unnecessary admissions, and facilitate early discharge when admissions occur. The Pfizer approach similarly targets those identified as being at highest need, using telephone case management to supplement existing services.

The NHS Institute for Innovation and Improvement (2006) provides the following information relating to evaluation of these approaches. Most information about the effects of Kaiser, Evercare and Pfizer is drawn from the USA. Evercare has been implemented with nine Primary Care Trusts in England and a national evaluation found that this model effectively identifies vulnerable older people, helps to provide preventive health care, and has the potential to organise care around people's needs. Nine other Primary Care Trusts are applying the Kaiser model, focusing on reducing hospital admissions by integrating services, with case studies suggesting some positive benefits. Another primary care trust is working with Pfizer to implement their InformaCare® model for chronic disease management. Although Kaiser and Pfizer have evaluated positively in the USA reducing hospital admissions and improving co-ordination of care no detailed information about outcomes from these service delivery models in the UK was identified.

The Strengths Model

The Strengths Model was developed in the early 1980s as an alternative to 'traditional' case management in mental health. It has been proposed that this model, drawn from social service perspectives, may be applied to service delivery in long-term care and other care for people with long-term conditions. The Strengths Model focuses on helping people and communities discover and develop their own talents, capacity and interests, and on connecting them with the resources they need to achieve their goals. Although the NHS Institute for Innovation and Improvement (2005) noted that there is evidence that the Strengths Model can improve satisfaction and quality of life in mental health, no studies of the effectiveness of this approach as a broader framework for chronic care service delivery were identified.

In a similar concept is the Adaptive Practice Model, the aim of this model being to encourage people with long-term conditions and their families to share decision-making responsibility with physicians. Again no studies of the effectiveness of this model for people with long-term conditions were identified by the NHS Institute for Innovation and Improvement (2005).

Guided care

Another emerging US service delivery model designed for older people with multiple chronic conditions is also being tested, with some reports suggesting that this model may improve quality of life and reduce health care resource use. This model is similar to the community matron role in the NHS and involves a specifically trained guided care nurse collaborating with primary care physicians to provide the following services for a target population of 40–60 people identified as high risk:

- comprehensive assessment and care planning
- 'best practices' for chronic conditions
- self-management
- healthy lifestyles
- coordinating care
- informing and supporting the family
- accessing community resources.

PACE Model

The final model reviewed is the Program of All-Inclusive Care for the Elderly (PACE), another US model of service provision and financing that aims to reduce use of hospital and nursing home care. The key feature of this model is integration of acute and long-term care services focusing on frail, elderly people with multiple problems attending day centres, allowing them to receive care from a single service organisation. The NHS Institute for Innovation and Improvement (2005) notes that this model is one of a number of similar health insurance provider initiatives in the USA but was selected for inclusion in the review, as it has been better documented than most. Little high-quality evidence was identified regarding its effectiveness, although numerous descriptive assessments were located. One comparative analysis suggested that PACE reduced hospital admissions compared to usual care, but increased the use of nursing homes.

The NHS Institute for Innovation and Improvement (2005) notes that the examples it provides are just a few of the thousands of service delivery models currently being implemented worldwide. The selected examples described merely illustrate that service delivery models tend to focus on selected components of broad chronic care frameworks. Although evaluations of individual services are available there is no clear evidence that one particular service delivery model is more effective than another. Further examples of frameworks used in selected countries, including the USA, Europe, Canada, New Zealand, Australia and Asia, are available from the full review document.

KEY POINTS

- Chronic diseases/long-term conditions can be controlled, not cured.
- Both incidence and prevalence of chronic diseases/long-term conditions are set to increase, attributable in part to an ageing population.
- Health policy, internationally, nationally and locally, is increasingly focused on effective management of chronic disease/long-term conditions.
- The Chronic Care Model and the related Innovative Care for Chronic Conditions Model are the most common frameworks for conceptualising effective components of care for people with long-term conditions.
- There is limited high-quality evidence about the impact of the effectiveness of any individual model, although there is evidence that components of the Chronic Care Model can improve quality of care and resource use.

FURTHER AREAS TO CONSIDER

- What is the local policy in your area regarding management of chronic disease/long-term conditions?
- Is this policy being guided by a national or local initiative?
- Have any specific service delivery models of care, for example, Evercare, been adopted in your locality?
- What system(s) have been put in place in your own practice area to ensure that the specific needs of people with chronic disease/long-term conditions are being met?
- What evaluation methods have been employed to determine the effectiveness of any approach that has been employed?

CHAPTER 2

PHYSICAL, PSYCHOLOGICAL AND PSYCHOSOCIAL IMPACT OF LIVING WITH A LONG-TERM CONDITION AND SOCIAL INFLUENCES ON HEALTH

OVERVIEW

This section reviews the current research looking at the impact that the diagnosis of a long-term condition can have on someone's life, including some of the physical, psychological and psychosocial effects of living with a long-term condition (LTC), both general and condition specific. Social and cultural influences on health are discussed, along with the importance of involving families and carers in care planning.

INTRODUCTION

Living with an LTC impacts on individuals in a number of ways, ranging from increased visits to the hospital/GP and dealing with complex medical regimes, to financial difficulties and social isolation from friends and family. A BMJ (2000, p. 526) editorial sums up the difference between acute and chronic disease as follows:

> With acute disease the treatment aims to return to normal. With chronic disease, the patient's life is irreversibly changed. Neither the disease nor its consequences are static. They interact to create illness patterns requiring continuous and complex management.

Living with an LTC is not just about living with the impact on physical health; LTCs are associated with depression and other psychological impacts on health. In addition, LTCs have a wider-reaching social impact, affecting every part of an individual's life including family relationships, employment and everyday socialisation. Having an LTC can limit an individual's ability to go to work or school or even take care of his or her own day-to-day physical needs. The DoH (2008b) notes that at all ages, people with an LTC affecting their day-to-day activities are twice as likely to be out of employment as those without LTCs. It is not only the individual with the LTC who is affected; caring for someone with an LTC can also have an impact on health. Rees *et al.* (2001) reviewed the impact of chronic disease on the quality of life of carers and concluded that partners who are carers also face numerous difficulties including:

- fear of the future;
- depression and/or anxiety;
- deterioration in partner relationship and/or sex life;
- concern about suffering of patient;
- implications of the care-giving role on their own health;
- fatigue/sleep deprivation;
- social disruption – either through looking after spouse or being unwilling to attend social functions alone;
- financial difficulties – patient and/or partner unable to continue working, expense of private care and adaptations to home.

(adapted from Rees *et al.* 2001)

This chapter will explore some of the physical, psychological and social impacts of living with an LTC for individuals, their families and carers.

PHYSICAL IMPACT

As noted in Chapter 1, LTCs or chronic illnesses cover a range of conditions: diabetes, cardiovascular disease (CVD) including heart disease, stroke and other diseases of the heart and circulation such as hypertension, congestive heart failure and peripheral vascular disease (PVD), chronic kidney disease (CKD), respiratory conditions such as asthma and chronic obstructive pulmonary disease (COPD), musculoskeletal conditions such as arthritis and osteoporosis, neurological conditions such as epilepsy, multiple sclerosis, Parkinson's and motor neurone disease (MND), skin disorders such as psoriasis, genetic conditions such as cystic fibrosis and muscular dystrophy, as well as certain mental conditions such as schizophrenia and dementia. This list is merely an example of the better-known conditions and is by no means conclusive. Indeed, the World Health Organisation (WHO) (2002b) expanded definition suggests that chronic conditions should not be viewed conventionally (limited to heart disease, diabetes, asthma), considered in isolation, or as disparate disorders but should include:

- non-communicable conditions
- persistent communicable conditions
- long-term mental disorders
- ongoing physical/structural impairments.

(WHO 2002b)

The WHO (2002b) also notes that physical disability or 'structural problems' including blindness or amputation are often the result of improper prevention or management of chronic conditions. The physical effects of all LTCs may include pain, disability, and change in the condition itself that can result in hospitalisation or more intensive care requirements, in addition to the potential development of both short- and long-term complications. The Department of Health (DoH) (2008b) notes that the 30 per cent of the population in England who say they suffer from an LTC use disproportionately more primary and secondary care services, accounting for 52 per cent of all GP appointments, 65 per cent of all outpatient appointments and 72 per cent of all inpatient bed days. However, although pain, disability and complications can be common side effects of a number of LTCs, many of the physical effects are condition specific. It would be impractical to attempt to describe the physical conditions and complications associated with all LTCs. This section will instead provide an overview of some of the physical effects associated with the more prevalent LTCs mentioned previously.

Diabetes mellitus

The prevalence of diabetes mellitus ranges worldwide from an average 3.66 per cent of the population in the UK in 2007 to 30.7 per cent of the population in the South Pacific island of Nauru (International Diabetes Federation (IDF) 2007). A diagnosis of diabetes is associated with significant potential short- and long-term complications (listed in Table 2.1), as well as the dietary and lifestyle changes required to achieve adequate control of the condition. For those diag- nosed with type 1 diabetes, there is the additional impact of adjusting to a lifestyle regime of insulin injections and regular blood glucose monitoring. For those diagnosed with type 2 diabetes, although initial treatment may involve diet/lifestyle changes only or a combination of diet and oral hypoglycaemic medication, many people progress to eventual treatment with insulin injections.

The short-term complications of diabetes mellitus include the life- threatening disorders of diabetic ketoacidosis (DKA) and hyperosmolar non- ketotic acidosis (HONK), as well as hypoglycaemia. DKA is a life-threatening complication of diabetes requiring emergency medical treatment; about 20 per

Table 2.1 Complications of diabetes mellitus

Short-term (acute) complications
Diabetic ketoacidosis (DKA)
Hyperosmolar non-ketotic acidosis (HONK)
Hypoglycaemia

Long-term (chronic) complications
Microvascular
Retinopathy
Nephropathy
Neuropathy

Macrovascular
Cardiovascular disease (CVD)
Peripheral vascular/arterial disease (PVD/PAD)
Diabetic foot (associated with PVD/PAD and/or neuropathy)

cent of cases are seen in undiagnosed type 1 diabetes, with the rest of the cases either associated with infection, other illnesses, cardiovascular disease, inadequate insulin use or unknown causes. It is much more common in younger people, particularly females; mortality rates vary from 1 to 10 per cent and are linked with case mix and management expertise (Patient UK 2006). HONK is more commonly seen in older people with type 2 diabetes. It occurs through a combination of intercurrent illness, dehydration and an inability to take normal medication due to illness. Like DKA it is a potentially life-threatening condition, characterised by severe hyperglycaemia and marked serum hyperosmolarity, but without evidence of severe ketosis due to the presence of basal insulin secretion. Patients normally present as extremely ill with signs of gross dehydration and require emergency medical treatment; mortality rate is 10 to 20 per cent (Patient UK 2008).

Hypoglycaemia is more common, but also easier to treat, providing that the person with diabetes is made aware of the symptoms and what to do. It can affect people with diabetes taking insulin and also those taking certain oral hypo-glycaemic medication. Treatment is simple and involves the person taking a fast-acting carbohydrate, followed up by a longer-acting carbohydrate (Diabetes UK 2006). However, if left untreated it can lead to unconsciousness requiring treatment by intramuscular glucagon (given by a trained user) or intravenous glucose (given by a health professional). Some people with diabetes may suffer with problematic hypoglycaemia or hypoglycaemia unawareness (NICE 2004b). Hypoglycaemic brain damage may also occur if hypoglycaemia is not treated correctly (NICE 2004b).

The potential long-term complications of diabetes include diabetic retinopathy causing deterioration in vision which can lead to eventual loss of vision; neuropathy which can cause numerous physical effects such as erectile dysfunction (ED), muscle wasting, reduced neurological sensation, foot deformi-ties and gastric disturbances; chronic kidney disease that can progress to end stage renal failure and CVD including heart disease, stroke and peripheral vascular disease which can lead to limb amputation. Diabetes is currently the leading cause of vision loss in adults of working age (20 to 65 years) in industrialised countries, the leading cause of non-traumatic limb amputation and the largest cause of kidney failure in developed countries, responsible for huge dialysis costs (IDF 2007). People with diabetes are five times more likely to develop CVD than those without diabetes and are as much at risk of having a myocardial infarction (MI) as those who have already had one (Diabetes UK 2006). Effective management and education can reduce the risk of both short- and long-term complications.

Cardiovascular disease

Cardiovascular disease is an umbrella term for all diseases of the heart and circulation, involving coronary heart disease, cerebrovascular disease and peripheral vascular/arterial disease; physical effects vary depending on the diagnosis. Risk factors for CVD include: smoking, hypertension, hyperlipidaemia, physical inactivity, being overweight or obese, having a diagnosis of diabetes and having a family history of heart disease. Physical effects of CVD range from the pain or tightness in the chest, arm, neck or jaw associated with angina, to the crushing pain, heaviness or chest tightness that can be the first sign of a myocardial infarction (British Heart Foundation 2008). People with angina need to learn to recognise the types of activity that may initiate an angina attack, how to treat it and how to distinguish between angina and the chest pain associated with a myocardial infarction. Cardiac rehabilitation programmes aim to assist people recovering from a cardiac event such as myocardial infarction or heart surgery and provide structured programmes of exercise and support, with multi-disciplinary input, to maximise recovery.

Heart failure can be associated with a previous myocardial infarction or may be a result of other conditions such as hypertension, cardiomyopathy or cardiac valve disease. Physical effects of heart failure include tiredness, breath-lessness, and swollen feet and ankles. People suffering with heart failure may find it difficult to take part in their normal day-to-day activities. Looking after someone with heart failure can be physically and emotionally demanding for carers. Heart support groups can help provide support, as well as appropriate treatment and self-help plans.

Cerebrovascular disease can lead to stroke, trans-ischaemic attacks or dementia. Strokes are not only the third most common cause of death in the UK, they are also the leading cause of severe disability, with more than 250,000 people in the UK living with disabilities caused by stroke (Stroke Association 2008). The Stroke Association provides a guide to some of the common problems associated with stroke. These include:

- weakness, clumsiness or paralysis (hemiplegia) usually affecting one side of the body
- spasticity of the muscles or joints
- loss of balance
- swallowing difficulties (dysphagia)
- extreme fatigue
- speech and communication difficulties (dysphasia)
- visual difficulties
- perception and interpretation difficulties
- reduced concentration and memory
- mood swings
- reduced sensation
- pain.

(adapted from Stroke Association 2008)

The Stroke Association also notes that although some of these problems may improve with time, improvement is often very gradual, and many survivors of stroke are left with significant long-term disability.

Peripheral vascular or *peripheral arterial disease* (PAD) is associated with significant pain and poor quality of life; symptoms can range from stage II, intermittent claudication (pain on walking relieved by rest), to stage III, rest and nocturnal pain, to stage IV, necrosis and gangrene. Pain is usually in the calves of the leg but may be in the thigh or buttock, and people with PAD may also suffer with cold or numb toes or feet and/or sores on toes, feet or legs that fail to heal. Patients with PAD, even in the absence of myocardial infarction or ischaemic stroke, have approximately the same relative risk of death from cardiovascular causes as do patients with a history of coronary or cerebro-vascular disease (SIGN 2006).

Chronic kidney disease

CKD is categorised into five stages, determined by measures of both estimated glomerular filtration rate and other renal tests or indicators, for example haematuria or proteinurea, structurally abnormal kidneys or genetic diagnosis of kidney disease:

- CKD stage 1 indicates normal kidney function but some signs of kidney disease.
- CKD stage 2 is mildly reduced kidney function.
- CKD stage 3 is a moderate reduction in kidney function.
- CKD stage 4 is a severe reduction in kidney function.
- CKD stage 5 is established kidney failure, when dialysis or a kidney transplant may be needed.

(adapted from Renal Association 2007)

Although the early stages of CKD should not cause any physical side effects, people diagnosed at this stage will need careful monitoring of blood pressure, blood sugar (to detect for diabetes if not previously diagnosed) and lipid levels, as risk of cardiovascular events and death is significantly increased even at this stage (Renal Association 2007). However, for those with more severe CKD cardiovascular risk is greatly increased, with a serious possibility that worsening kidney disease could lead to serious illness or death without treatment at stage 4. Dialysis or transplantation is often required at stage 5 (end-stage renal failure). Physical signs of stages 4 and 5 can include tiredness, loss of appetite, itchiness, swollen ankles, high blood pressure, reduced sex drive and frequent nocturia (EdRen 2006). People with stage 4 or 5 CKD are encouraged to live normal lifestyles but activities such as holidays may need careful planning to fit in with treatment plans.

Respiratory conditions

Asthma

Asthma is a chronic inflammatory condition of the airways where the airways are hyper-responsive and constrict easily in response to a wide range of stimuli. Physical effects of poorly controlled asthma include coughing, wheezing, chest tightness and shortness of breath (Clinical Knowledge Summaries (CKS) 2007a). More than 1,400 people died of asthma in the UK in 2002. On average, one person dies of asthma every seven hours; in addition, asthma accounts for one out of every 250 deaths worldwide (CKS 2007a). Asthma can lead to respiratory complications such as respiratory failure and status asthmaticus (repeated asthma attacks without respite, or non-response to appropriate treatment), as well as growth and pubertal delay and impaired quality of life including: fatigue, underperformance and time off school and work (CKS 2007a).

The Asthma UK Cymru (2008) report *A Quarter of a Million Voices ... and Counting* notes that people living in deprived areas are most likely to feel that their asthma is out of control and limits their lives and to have lower expectations of how their asthma treatment can help their condition. The report also notes that despite improvements in asthma treatment and medication, 24 per cent of people with asthma feel there is nothing they can do to limit their asthma symptoms, with one in seven feeling that the condition has a negative impact on how other people see them. Keeping asthma under control both prevents symptoms and exacerbations and reduces morbidity and mortality.

Chronic obstructive pulmonary disease

COPD is a term used for a number of conditions causing long-term lung damage and subsequent difficulty in breathing including chronic bronchitis and emphysema. Symptoms of COPD include cough, phlegm and shortness of breath. COPD can also lead to feelings of anxiety, resulting in people with COPD limiting their activities which in turn leads to further breathlessness due to reduced fitness levels. Depending on the severity of the condition symptoms can be mild and only occur at certain times, during winter or after a cold (British Lung Foundation 2007). In severe cases shortness of breath can affect all aspects of daily activities, causing the individual to have problems with mobility, sleeping, eating and talking as well as breathing. This may necessitate the long-term use of oxygen, which can further restrict normal daily activities of living. Mortality due to COPD is still increasing; it is currently the fourth leading cause of death worldwide and the WHO (2006a) predicts that death rates globally from COPD will rise from 4.8 per cent in 2002 to 7.9 per cent by 2030. In addition, in terms of the proportion of total disability adjusted life years lost (DALYs) COPD is set to rise in the ranking from eleventh in 2002 to fourth in 2030 (WHO 2006a).

COPD was until recently often misdiagnosed and subsequently poorly managed. The NICE (2004d) guideline on COPD set out clear recommendations for both diagnosis and treatment of the disease, and the inclusion of COPD in the Quality and Outcomes Framework (QOF) in the UK new General Medical Services (nGMS) Contract (BMA/NHS Confederation 2003) has resulted in improved care for sufferers, particularly in primary care. Halpin (2008) suggests, however, that there is evidence that, in contrast with asthma, COPD is still under-treated by primary care physicians, particularly in the early stages of the disease. He also notes that reduced health status/health-related quality of life, measured by standardised approved questionnaires, is gaining increasing recognition as a predictor of mortality, as well as the impact of frequency and severity of exacerbations on both morbidity and mortality. Early and correct diagnosis, smoking cessation, appropriate treatment, preventing and treating exacerbations and pulmonary rehabilitation involving exercise and education can help prevent deterioration and improve quality of life.

Musculoskeletal conditions

Arthritis

Nine million people in the UK suffer from some sort of arthritis (inflammation of the joints) (Arthritis Care 2008), and in Wales alone it is the most commonly reported chronic condition. In the USA arthritis is the most common cause of disability, limiting the activities of nearly 19 million adults (National Centre for Chronic Disease Prevention and Health Promotion 2008). In Australia, 3.85 million adults are affected and Arthritis Australia (2008) notes that this has a significant effect on the economy in terms of loss of earnings and lost production.

There are over 200 forms of arthritis; two of the most common forms are osteoarthritis, where the cartilage between the bone degenerates, leading to painful rubbing of bone on bone and potential joint misalignment, and rheumatoid arthritis, where the body's immune system attacks and destroys the joint, causing pain, swelling and reduction of movement. Other common forms of rheumatic or musculoskeletal conditions that fall under the arthritis umbrella include gout, ankylosing spondylitis, fibromyalgia and systemic lupus erythematosis. Pain, stiffness and fatigue are common side effects of all arthritic conditions, as well as loss of strength and movement in inflamed joints (Arthritis Care 2008). These arthritis-related problems can result in joint weakness, instability and deformities that can interfere with common daily activities, including walking, driving and food preparation (Arthritis Australia 2008). Arthritis can affect people of all ages, including children, with about one in a thousand children developing juvenile idiopathic arthritis.

Osteoporosis

Osteoporosis is a disease characterised by low bone mass and microarchitectural deterioration of bone tissue, with a consequent increase in bone fragility and susceptibility to fracture (CKS 2006c). Along with falls, osteoporosis is a key risk factor for fracture. Fractures can occur at any site but are most common at the spine, wrist and hip, with hip fracture the most common serious injury after a fall. Within the UK approximately 14,000 people die each year as a result of hip fracture, with 50 per cent of survivors no longer able to live independently. Hip fracture is also associated with other complications such as deep vein thrombosis, pulmonary embolism and pneumonia. Not all osteoporotic fractures are related to falls. Only 25 per cent of vertebral fractures are associated with falls, the rest occurring due to the underlying bone fragility. Following one vertebral fracture the risk of another is increased sevenfold. Many people with vertebral fractures are left with chronic back pain, and multiple vertebral fractures can lead to stooped posture and loss of height. In addition, people who have had a fragility fracture are at risk of further fractures and increased mortality (CKS 2006c). The increased mortality rate associated with osteoporosis is related to the complications associated with fracture, rather than the disease process itself.

Long-term neurological conditions

The *National Service Framework* (DoH 2005d) defines a long-term neurological condition as a condition that results from disease of, injury or damage to the body's nervous system (brain, spinal cord and/or their peripheral nerve connections), which will affect the individual and his or her family in one way or another for the rest of his or her life. Taken together, long-term neurological conditions account for 20 per cent of acute hospital admissions and are the third most common reason for seeing a GP, with an estimated 350,000 people across the UK needing help with daily living owing to a neurological condition and 850,000 people caring for someone with a neurological condition (DoH 2005d). The NSF further categorises long-term neurological conditions as:

- Sudden-onset conditions such as acquired brain injury or spinal cord injury, followed by a partial recovery.
- Intermittent and unpredictable conditions; for example, epilepsy, certain types of headache or early multiple sclerosis, where relapses and remissions lead to marked variation in the care needed.
- Progressive conditions; for example, motor neurone disease, Parkinson's disease or later stages of multiple sclerosis, where progressive deterioration in neurological function leads to increasing dependence on help and care from others.
- Stable neurological conditions, but with changing needs due to development or ageing; for example, post-polio syndrome or cerebral palsy in adults.

(DoH 2005d, p. 9)

Depending on the condition and its progression, long-term neurological conditions can be associated with a number of problems including:

- Physical or motor problems (including incontinence, paralysis, fatigue)
- Sensory problems (including hearing, pain or vision loss)
- Cognitive/behavioural problems
- Communication difficulties.

(DoH 2005d, pp. 10–11)

Epilepsy

Epilepsy is a condition characterised by recurrent, unprovoked seizures, with an epileptic seizure defined as a brief disturbance of consciousness, behaviour, emotion, motor function or sensation that is due to abnormal electrical discharge in the brain (CKS 2006b). Epilepsy is the most common serious neurological condition in the world, with one in every 131 people in the UK suffering from it. There are different types and causes of epilepsy and it affects all ages, races and social classes. Within the UK people with epilepsy are not allowed to hold a driving licence until they have been seizure free for one year. The National Society for Epilepsy (2007) advises that if seizures are controlled, epilepsy should not stop anyone leading a full and active life; however, those who continue to have seizures may need to consider measures to ensure their safety, for example having a stair guard in their home. Following a seizure a person with epilepsy may feel drowsy, bite his or her tongue or suffer from aching limbs. Severity of seizures can vary from a trance-like state for a few seconds or minutes to loss of consciousness and severe convulsions (CKS 2006b). Physical injuries can occur because of seizures and about 500 deaths a year occur in the UK due to sudden unexpected death in epilepsy (SUDEP). Status epilepticus, a seizure that lasts for more than thirty minutes or repeated seizures, is another severe potential complication of epilepsy that can lead to brain damage if not treated correctly (CKS 2006b).

Skin conditions

Skin conditions cover a wide range, from short and self-limiting to long-term conditions that can be treated but not cured. The intention of including them in this chapter is not to provide a comprehensive overview, but purely to note that some long-term skin conditions can cause significant physical effects, including pain, discomfort and potential complications. *Eczema*, for example, can present as:

- mild: with areas of dry skin and/or infrequent itching;
- moderate: with areas of dry skin, frequent itching and redness;
- severe: causing redness, with or without excoriation, extensive skin thickening, bleeding, oozing, cracking and alteration of pigmentation.

(CKS 2008a)

Psoriasis, which affects 2 to 3 per cent of the population of the UK, also varies greatly in severity, from small, red, flaky, crusty patches that come and go, to more severe forms that may require intensive medical or nursing care. Between 10 per cent and 20 per cent of people with psoriasis develop psoriatic arthritis, which causes general tiredness, tenderness, pain and swelling over tendons, swollen fingers and toes, stiffness, pain, throbbing, swelling and tenderness in one or more joints, reduced range of movement and nail changes (Psoriasis Association 2008). As with all LTCs, individuals suffering from long-term skin conditions need appropriate management, support and advice to help them manage their conditions and reduce physical symptoms.

PAUSE FOR REFLECTION

Think about your own lifestyle: what would you have to change if you developed an LTC?

This section has provided an overview of some of the physical problems associated with living with an LTC. It is clear that the onset of an LTC can bring with it significant physical changes, and subsequent lifestyle adjustment requirements, in addition to an increased risk of mortality. Health care professionals through regular monitoring and review can assist people with LTCs in making these lifestyle adjustments and ensure appropriate treatment and care plans are devised and instigated to maximise health and minimise side effects, relating to both the condition and treatment. People with LTCs should also be provided with information regarding appropriate charities that can offer help and advice specific to each LTC.

PSYCHOLOGICAL/PSYCHOSOCIAL IMPACT

> Depression refers to a wide range of mental health problems characterised by the absence of a positive affect (a loss of interest and enjoyment in ordinary things and experiences), low mood and a range of associated emotional, cognitive, physical and behavioural symptoms.
>
> (NICE 2004a, p. 13)

Depression affects an estimated 10 per cent of the adult population. By the year 2020, it is estimated that depression will be surpassed only by heart disease in terms of the disability it causes with substantial personal, social and economic impacts (WHO 2002b). Although depression on its own is considered to be an LTC, depression has also been noted as a significant co-morbidity condition with other LTCs. As well as patients with LTCs being more likely to develop depression, it has also been suggested that people who are depressed are more likely to develop a physical LTC (Elder and Holmes 2002). Depression is frequently accompanied by anxiety symptoms but may occur on its own (NICE 2004a). Depression ranges greatly in severity, with symptoms including tearfulness, irritability, reduced sleep and appetite, pain, fatigue, lack of libido, lowered self-esteem and marked anxiety, and can lead to attempts at self-harm and suicide (NICE 2004a).

Lyons *et al.* (2006) in their report *Long-term Conditions and Depression*, undertaken for the Care Services Improvement Partnership (CSIP), note that depression, as a cause or consequence of physical illness, particularly diabetes, cardiovascular and cerebrovascular disease, may exacerbate the perceived severity of symptoms and distress and increase the utilisation of health services. Patients with cardiac disease and depression have been shown to be at increased risk of death; similarly, depressed people without cardiac disease have been shown to have increased risk of cardiac mortality (NICE 2004a). Lyons *et al.* (2006) summarise the key issues regarding the mental health component of LTCs as shown in Table 2.2.

Certain LTCs such as stroke result in not only complex physical consequences but psychological, emotional and social sequelae which are often

Table 2.2 Key issues

The mental health component of long-term conditions adversely impacts on:

- health outcomes
- disabilities
- health resource utilisation.

Medically unexplained symptoms are common.
Medically unexplained symptoms are a significant cause of disability and distress.
Medically unexplained symptoms are costly.

(adapted from Lyons *et al.* 2006, p.13)

deep-rooted (Thompson and Ryan 2008). A review of the psychosocial consequences of stroke carried out by Thompson and Ryan (2008, p. 178) suggested
a number of key consequences of stroke that impact on both individuals and
their spouses:

- Dependency – Over-solicitous care of the person with stroke
  fostering helplessness and dependency. Decline in social
  interaction can jeopardise spousal relationships.
- Loss of work – Associated loss of income, reduced social
  contact and changes in lifestyle can have detrimental effects on
  a stroke survivor's relationship with his or her partner.
- Fatigue – Lowers motivation, and interferes with physical
  functioning, work, family and social life.
- Decline in sexual activity – Many people experience a decline in
  sexual activity following a stroke. Psychological issues such as
  fear of a recurrent stroke, impaired self-esteem, changes in body
  image and a reluctance to discuss sexuality with a spouse are
  contributing factors.

Also noted in the review was that in a study utilising the European Brain Injury
Questionnaire, depressive mood, loneliness, cognitive difficulties and lack of
autonomy were the most frequent problems reported by stroke survivors.

Depression and disability have also been noted as predictors of mortality
in patients discharged from hospital following acute exacerbations of COPD
(Halpin 2008). Links between COPD, depression and anxiety have been well
documented (British Lung Foundation 2007) with the physical effects of living
with lung disease, such as tiredness, difficulty in sleeping and eating, self-
consciousness about coughing or needing to use oxygen and an inability to
participate in activities previously enjoyed resulting in depression. Many people
with COPD become anxious due to not feeling in control of their health. The
British Lung Foundation (2007) provides advice and guidance to encourage
people with COPD who are feeling anxious and/or depressed to seek help and
support.

PAUSE FOR REFLECTION

What services are you aware of to which you could refer someone who is suffering with anxiety and depression related to an LTC?

Numerous other LTCs are also linked with increased incidence of depression. Depression is thought to affect about half of all people with Parkinson's disease (National Collaborating Centre for Chronic Conditions (NCC-CC) 2006). Mayor (2007) makes the point that the diagnosis of mild depression can be difficult to make in Parkinson's disease because of the overlapping of motor symptoms with features of clinical depression. She also notes that depression is the single most important predictor of quality of life in Parkinson's disease, and can impair efforts to control symptoms and cause tension with carers. It has also been shown that depression is three times more likely in patients suffering from rheumatoid arthritis (Sheehy *et al.* 2006). In the UK the GMS contract (BMA/NHS Confederation 2003) has made some attempt to encourage practices to detect depression in patients with LTCs through the inclusion of two screening questions within the QOF:

- During the past month, have you been feeling down, depressed or hopeless?
- During the past month, have you often been bothered by having little interest or pleasure in doing things?

A positive answer to either of these questions is followed up with referral to a GP for further screening, using one of three validated screening tools: the Patient Health Questionnaire, Hospital Anxiety and Depression Scale or the Beck Depression Inventory Second Edition. An appropriate treatment plan should then be put into place if indicated. However, these questions are only aimed at patients attending for diabetes and coronary heart disease reviews and do not include any of the other LTCs. NICE (2004a) suggests screening in those with a past history of depression, significant physical illness, especially if it causes disability, and other mental health problems like dementia.

This section has provided a brief overview of some of the potential psychological impacts on health for people with LTCs. Living with an LTC is clearly not just about living with the physical effects of illness. Health care providers should be aware of the signs and symptoms of depression and anxiety, utilise suitable screening tools and instigate appropriate programmes of care in conjunction with mental health professionals to ensure that people with LTCs receive appropriate treatment and support.

SOCIAL INFLUENCES ON HEALTH

It is well established that health status is largely determined by a person's social environment and vice versa. Policy documents in recent decades have shifted the emphasis from a focus on individual responsibility for health to a more holistic approach that includes socioeconomic, environmental and cultural influences. The biomedical model of health has been dominant in Western societies since the great advances in science and technology of the nineteenth and twentieth centuries, and is associated with the increasing power of the medical profession. The main features of the medical model of health are listed below.

- The mind and body are separate.
- The body acts like a machine that can be 'fixed'.
- Doctors are like engineers, mending broken parts.
- Health is absence of disease.
- Psychosocial and environmental factors are largely ignored.

(Nettleton 2006)

PAUSE FOR REFLECTION

The main cause of sickness and death in the nineteenth century was infectious disease. The course of the twentieth century saw a decline in morbidity and an increase in life expectancy. How much of the improvement in health was attributable to medical progress?

Sociologists argue that the effect of advances in science and technology is marginal in comparison to improvements in living conditions and standards, nutrition and hygiene. In addition, some sociologists cite the harmful effects of medical interventions or iatrogenesis as a consequence (Illich 1976). In clinical terms, this means that some treatments and drugs can have harmful side effects. In social terms, medical interventions can result in a dependence on medical science and a loss of coping strategies. Sociologists purport that health and illness are social constructs and are determined by social forces such as class (Nettleton 2006).

People suffering from LTCs are more likely to be poor and living in deprived areas than the general population, and this is a factor that is included in the census and population-based statistics such as indices of deprivation (ONS 2005). Indeed, a social class gradient can be attached to nearly every cause of morbidity and mortality. Recent policy directives have attempted to address this issue both from the global perspective and nationally. The WHO in its various charters and declarations has emphasised the relevance of inequalities in health, empowerment and sustainable communities (WHO 1978, 1986, 1991). Similarly, UK government policies since 1997 have echoed these themes by tackling inequalities in health, working in partnership with clients and other professionals, focusing on primary care, public health, and prevention and improving quality being top of the political agenda (DoH 1997, 1999; WAG 2001, 2005).

PAUSE FOR REFLECTION

Recent statistics from 2001 to 2003 reveal that the difference in male life expectancy at birth between Glasgow City (the lowest at 69.1) and East Dorset (the highest at 80.1) remains eleven years (ONS 2004).

Individual determinants of health:

- genetic factors
- age
- gender
- ethnicity
- lifestyle factors
- family
- friends and neighbours.

Social determinants of health:

- income
- housing and living conditions
- employment and working conditions
- education
- culture
- health services
- water and sanitation
- access to healthy foods
- environment.

(adapted from Dahlgren and Whitehead 1991)

Individual determinants of health

These lists are not exhaustive and there is inevitably overlap between the two. Some individual factors are fixed and cannot be changed such as genetics, age, ethnicity and gender (in most cases). Recently, there has been a greater emphasis on *genetic factors*, for instance relating to the risk of developing breast cancer, and some LTCs are strongly associated with family history and may require genetic counselling and intervention.

Age has an obvious impact on LTCs and the increase in prevalence has been closely linked to demographic changes and the ageing population. The development of illness can be devastating at any age, causing social isolation, stigma and depression. In younger people, who are sensitive to body image and peer pressure, the development of an LTC can affect self-esteem and confidence, and may cause interruption of study and work patterns. Concordance with medication such as using inhalers for asthma may be avoided in order to be less conspicuous. Blaxter (1990) identified different attitudes to health through the lifespan, with young men emphasising physical fitness, while older people stress being able to function and peace of mind as important.

Some patterns of LTCs are *gender* specific such as certain cancers and other conditions that are more prevalent in men than in women and vice versa. Feminist writers emphasise the position of women in society and how this affects their everyday life (Oakley 1993). Women in employment still tend to be lower paid and part time, with fewer privileges or opportunities for promotion than men, despite four decades of supposed equal opportunities (Government Equalities Office 2008). This has an impact on people with LTCs as women are more likely to become informal carers than men and are more likely to suffer mental health problems as a result (ONS 2002).

The pattern of LTCs in *ethnic minority* groups may be determined by genetic or cultural factors. There is a higher prevalence of diabetes in the South Asian population, for example, and cultural attitudes towards diet could be responsible for the increased or decreased prevalence of heart disease (Chowdhury 2003). Institutional racism means that people from ethnic minority groups tend to have lower-paid jobs and live in poorer areas while fear of racist attack can lead to social isolation, anxiety and depression. In addition, access to health services may be hindered by language difficulties (McKenzie 2003).

Individual lifestyle factors have been given considerable credence in determining health status and can be considered in the light of political ideology. The Conservative government in 1992, for example, issued a policy document that was heavily criticised for 'victim blaming', that is, for placing responsibility for health on individual behaviour and ignoring the wider social determinants (DoH 1992). Behaviour change is a very complex issue and continues to be hotly debated, with certain treatments being withheld from people who are considered unworthy (Donnelly 2008). This can have a stigmatising effect for those suffering from certain LTCs: COPD and its links to smoking, and type 2 diabetes and its possible links to obesity are examples.

PAUSE FOR REFLECTION

Have you ever tried to change any aspect of your lifestyle? What were the factors that assisted you and what were the barriers to change?

Family, community and social networks are extremely important in considering the social impact of LTCs. The onset of illness has a profound effect on the family members of the patient, not only in their possible role as carers but in their sensitivity to the possible stigmatising effects of certain illnesses. Recent decades have seen the breakdown of the traditional extended family and community. High levels of divorce, single parenthood, geographical and social mobility and the concentration of families with multiple social problems in certain areas such as sink estates have had an impact. Fear of crime and vandalism causes anxiety that can lead to mental health problems and physical manifestations (Nettleton 2006).

Social determinants of health

As previously stated, social class impacts greatly upon health status. This is determined broadly by occupation and affects many other aspects of life. The most obvious is *income*. People with LTCs are more likely to be poor in the first place as poverty is a major determinant of health (Acheson 1998). This is further exacerbated by the fact that they may be forced to give up employment or already be retired, and is compounded by the possibility of the carer also having to relinquish a paid wage, forcing him or her on to state benefits. Income determines many other aspects of lifestyle, particularly *housing* choices. Living conditions are very influential in health outcomes; for instance, cold and damp are associated with respiratory diseases. Those who have to spend more than 10 per cent of their income to adequately heat their homes are deemed to be in 'fuel poverty'. This is particularly relevant in the current situation as the price of fuel is rising and more people are likely to fall into this category. Every year in the UK, thousands die from 'excess winter deaths' as a result and many of them are likely to be LTC sufferers with limited mobility. Those who are housebound will need to heat their homes for longer periods during the day (DEFRA 2008).

In certain areas, access to services is also restricted. This applies to *health services* and evokes the 'Inverse care law' which states that those who are most in need of medical services are less likely to use them or to use them as effectively as those in less need (Tudor-Hart 1971). This has obvious repercussions for LTC sufferers who will need more frequent contact with health care professionals than the general population. Other services also fall into this bracket; transport may be inadequate and this is crucial to those who are unable to drive, and access to cheaper, *healthier foods* through supermarkets may also be difficult. This could be an important issue for people with type 2 diabetes and coronary heart disease (CHD) whose diet and possible control of obesity are contingent to their well-being.

PAUSE FOR REFLECTION

What factors influence your choices when buying food?

Those whose conditions allow them to maintain *employment* may find other issues come to the fore. Certain illnesses such as epilepsy or diabetes can be concealed if the person wishes and he or she may then feel in constant fear of 'being found out'. Employers and colleagues may be more sympathetic to certain illnesses than others and in any case frequent absences from work may be required for hospital and other appointments, which may be problematic. The acceptance is dependent on the person's access to the 'sick role', described by Parsons (1951), who contended that illness is a form of deviance that goes against the work ethic of capitalist society. Access to the sick role is granted by medical acceptance of the condition (Friedson 1970). Some LTCs may be linked to employment; for instance, 10 per cent of adult-onset asthma is caused by occupational factors such as inhaling chemicals (BTS/SIGN 2008). Stress is often associated with working practices but losing a job will usually result in loss of income and can also change a person's sense of identity and lower his or her self-esteem, often leading to mental health problems and an increased risk of suicide. Physical illness is also more prevalent (Centre for Economic Policy Research 2008).

Environmental factors are essential in determining health status. In the past in the UK, pollution, overcrowding and poor hygiene were responsible for deadly outbreaks of infectious diseases. Public health measures brought about massive improvements, shifting the main cause of mortality and morbidity to LTCs (Craig 2002). The effects of global warming are currently being widely debated through-out the world and are a huge challenge to all governments (DEFRA 2008). In the UK, basic amenities such as clean water and sanitation are taken for granted but in developing countries, lack of these amenities still causes thousands of deaths each year and is a serious indictment of everyone concerned (UNICEF 2007).

Social influences are critical in considering all aspects of health and are particularly relevant to those suffering from an LTC. This section has merely outlined some of the issues to be considered and is hopefully a starting point for further interest and study.

KEY POINTS

- Although people with LTCs can suffer from similar physical symptoms, such as pain and reduced mobility, many of the physical symptoms associated with individual LTCs are condition specific.
- As well as the more obvious physical impacts of living with an LTC, people with LTCs are also prone to psychological conditions such as anxiety and depression.
- When assessing the needs of a person with an LTC, social influences should also be taken into account and not considered in isolation.
- Individual determinants of health should be incorporated when planning appropriate health care.

FURTHER AREAS TO CONSIDER

- Are there any specific social factors influencing health in your area?
- How can you ensure that you include individual determinants of health when planning individual health care?
- What assessment are you using currently when assessing people with LTCs to screen for depression?

CHAPTER 3

CASE MANAGEMENT AND DISEASE-SPECIFIC CARE MANAGEMENT

OVERVIEW

The current policy emphasis is on moving patients out of acute care settings and providing care in the community. For patients with long-term conditions (LTCs) it has long been accepted that care should be provided in the primary care/community setting with a firm emphasis on self-care. People with LTCs use disproportionately more primary and secondary care services (DoH 2008b), a pattern that is set to increase with an ageing population. The role of the district nurse is currently under scrutiny with many areas adopting the community matron who manages a case load and works closely with patients to prevent unnecessary hospital admission. This chapter will explore the principles behind case management and disease-specific care management including new and existing nursing roles and the importance of multi-disciplinary team involvement.

INTRODUCTION

In Chapter 1 the guiding strategic and theoretical frameworks and policies relating to the care of individuals with LTCs were introduced. The aim of this chapter is to discuss in further detail the principles behind case management and disease-specific care management. Existing nursing roles, such as district nursing and practice nursing in meeting the needs of people with LTCs, will be reviewed, in addition to the community matron/advanced primary nurse role. The importance of adopting a team approach to care will also be discussed, appreciating the contribution made by numerous health care professionals in meeting the LTC care agenda.

Within the UK a key aspect of the National Health Service (NHS) and Social Care Long Term Conditions Model, based on the US Kaiser Permanente triangle of care management (DoH 2005c), is the three-tier triangle approach, stratifying patients in order to match them to appropriate packages of care. This three-tier approach involves:

> *Level 3*: Case management – requires the identification of the very high intensity users of unplanned secondary care. Care for these patients is to be managed using a community matron or other professional using a case management approach, to anticipate, co-ordinate and join up health and social care.

> *Level 2*: Disease-specific care management – This involves providing people who have a complex single need or multiple conditions with responsive, specialist services using multi-disciplinary teams and disease-specific protocols and pathways, such as the National Service Frameworks [NSF] and Quality and Outcomes Framework [QOF].

> *Level 1*: Supported self-care – collaboratively helping individuals and their carers to develop the knowledge, skills and confidence to care for themselves and their condition effectively.

> (DoH 2005c)

The self-care/self-management approach to care will be discussed in Chapter 4. This chapter will concentrate on reviewing existing and new methods of care, in addition to the nursing and health care roles that contribute to them, at levels 2 and 3: case management and disease-specific care management.

CASE MANAGEMENT

Definition and models

The term 'case management' originates from the USA where it was originally developed, with its roots in social care, as a method of 'delivering holistic individualized care, tailored to the needs of people with complex health and social care problems' (Hutt *et al.* 2004, p. 6). Initially instigated in the 1950s to provide care to patients with severe mental health problems, it was expanded for use with older people with complex health and social care needs, to both contain health care costs and coordinate services to reduce the need for institutional care (Drennan and Goodman 2004; Hutt *et al.* 2004). Definitions of case management include 'the process of planning, coordinating, managing and reviewing the care of an individual', with the aim being: 'to develop cost-effective and efficient ways of coordinating services in order to improve quality of life' (Hutt *et al.* 2004, p. 6). Reviewing types of case management approaches, Drennan and Goodman (2004) note that two types of case manager role may be adopted: the brokerage model (similar to the UK social worker model), where case managers hold the budget to finance user care packages, and the key worker extension model, which is closer to the approach historically used by district nurses in the UK, where the case manager both provides and coordinates services for the user.

Within the UK, England piloted the US nurse-led Evercare model, introduced in 2003 in nine Primary Care Trusts (PCTs), with the appointment of Advanced Primary Nurses (APNs), also referred to as community matrons, to take on the case management role. Apart from Evercare, other US service models, developed by Pfizer and Kaiser Permanente, have also been piloted in areas of the UK (see Chapter 1 for descriptions of these models). These models are by no means universal throughout the four countries of the UK, however. Wales, for example, has taken on different approaches in each locality, adopting a variety of diverse methods to take the practical aspects of the long-term conditions management agenda forward. This has included the development of LTC teams who support practice nurses and general practitioners (GPs) through the provision of educational updates, or who work with primary health care teams (PHCT) to assist them with managing more complex patients.

Community matrons

A community matron is described in the NHS plan (DoH 2004b, p. 34) as:

> An individual who is experienced, skilled and uses case management techniques with patients who make high use of health care services, with the ultimate aim of remaining at home longer with more choice about their health care.

The community matron/APN is expected to be an experienced nurse, already working in the NHS, who has a wide range of competencies. These include high-level assessment and clinical skills to meet physical, mental and social care needs; an ability to identify high-risk patients; to lead complex care coordination, including liaising and synchronising inputs from other agencies; to review and prescribe medications; to support self-care and independence and be highly visible to patients, their families and carers and seen as being in charge of their care (DoH 2005a). They manage the care of people with one or more LTCs, or who have a complex mix of medical and social problems and are intensive users of health care services, including frequent admissions to hospital. The intention behind the community matron role was that they would provide a more holistic approach to care, overseeing a caseload of up to 80 patients and coordinating health and social care provision with the overall aim of promoting maximum function, independence and improved quality of life. The role itself offers autonomy and independence to influence service delivery and maintain clinical credibility, while remaining closely involved with patient care.

It is important to note at this stage that nurses working in a range of roles in primary care, particularly district nurses, have always made significant contributions to the care of people with LTCs, specifically the elderly population, using case management techniques (Drennan and Goodman 2004). Indeed, following the evaluation of the initial Evercare pilot sites in England, While (2007) commented that the pilot programmes had made little significant impact on overall health care outcomes, including emergency admissions and bed days, and that community matrons cannot substitute for the district nursing work-force, whose service needs to be revitalised and retooled.

Worldwide, different approaches have been adopted. Australia, for exam-ple, has a case management society to advance the practice of case management and educate health care organisations, health care professionals and the public. Australia's policies are currently under review in light of recent governmental changes; however, the National Chronic Disease Strategy (NHPAC 2006) at the time of writing sets out a three-stage triangular approach to care, similar to that in the UK (Figure 3.1).

Services in Australia are being developed to improve care coordination for all those with LTCs, with plans to provide integration and continuity of prevention and care, through the use of care coordinators, to ensure that multi-disciplinary care plans are carried through and regularly reviewed. Access to appropriate services is seen as a priority, particularly for Aboriginal and Torres Strait Islander peoples, rural and remote communities and other underserviced population groups (NHPAC 2006). In New Zealand at the time of writing, a

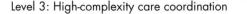

Level 3: High-complexity care coordination

Level 2: High-risk disease/care management

Level 1: 70–80 per cent chronic disease population – self-management support

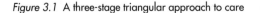

Figure 3.1 A three-stage triangular approach to care

Long Term Conditions Framework is in the process of being developed (Ministry of Health NZ 2008).

Effectiveness of case management

A King's Fund report (Hutt *et al.* 2004) examined the effectiveness of case management, drawing on studies mainly from the USA but also from Canada, Italy, Denmark and Scotland. The review focused particularly on the transferability of these models to the UK and identified a number of important issues. These included the variability of economic and regulatory environments between countries that can make it harder to reproduce patterns of utilisation and cost savings reported in other countries. Second, they noted that the differences in training and skills of the staff providing case management raised questions about the feasibility of transferring findings from the USA to the UK NHS, with many US nurse case managers trained to Masters level. Third, they noted that patient selection techniques are imprecise and do not always predict who may benefit most from case management. In addition, they emphasised that components of case management could duplicate other services offered by the NHS such as hospital outreach and community-based services. Overall the review concluded that there is limited evidence regarding the most effective types of case management. Where case management is being implemented the local NHS providers need to be clear about the needs of the population at whom it is aimed; discuss whether existing services can be adapted; develop case management in close collaboration with social care providers; ensure that adequate systems are in place for those with less severe illness, and evaluate initiatives in terms of both their impact on the health service and patient satisfaction (Hutt *et al.* 2004).

The final report of the evaluation of Evercare pilot sites in the UK (Boaden *et al.* 2006) indicated a contradiction between the qualitative and quantitative findings. The qualitative findings suggested that both patients and carers experienced a high level of satisfaction with the service. They particularly valued the psychological support; the rapid response in times of crisis, and the ability of the APNs to monitor medications, organise prescriptions, explain LTCs, investigations and treatments, and to provide advocacy for patients. The APNs reported many examples where they had altered medication and coordinated care to avoid hospital admissions, improve quality of life and reduce fragmentation of services. However, the quantitative evaluation showed no significant effect on emergency admissions, emergency bed days or mortality, for either the high-risk groups or the general over-65 population. The report concluded that Evercare provided a workable model of case management, which was popular with APNs, patients and carers. It also noted that adoption of this system provided patients and carers with frequency of contact, regular monitoring and knowledge of referral procedures: options that had not previously been provided. However, no overall evidence of systematic redesign of care was identified and it was noted that this would need to be addressed in future if hospital admissions were to be reduced.

PAUSE FOR REFLECTION

Has case management been introduced in your area, and has it had an impact on overall health outcomes? If you are a case manager, what educational preparation did you receive for the role? Did you feel adequately prepared?

Practicalities of case management

If a case management strategy is to be adopted, the identification of suitable patients/clients is essential. In order to identify which patients/clients would be most suitable for case management, those who present with the most complex conditions and are considered vulnerable or at risk of hospitalisation or requiring institutionalised care need to be identified by the appropriate health and social care organisation (DoH 2005c). In the UK a number of software tools have been developed that can assist with this process. Criteria for selection include the following:

- number of hospital admissions and lengths of stay;
- co-morbidity (number of medical and other problems that a patient may have);
- number of medications a patient is prescribed;
- number of GP consultations;
- other high-risk factors (such as living alone/unsupported).

(adapted from DoH 2005c)

Additional criteria used in the Evercare pilots included:

- Recent exacerbation or decompensation of chronic illness
- Recent falls (more than two falls in two months)
- Recent bereavement and at risk of medical decline
- Cognitively impaired, living alone, medically unstable and high-intensity social service package.

(DoH 2005c, p. 16)

Drennan and Goodman (2004) suggest that case management has the core activities at individual patient level listed in Table 3.1.

Table 3.1 Core activities at individual patient level

- Identification of individuals likely to benefit from case management
- Assessment of the individual's problems and need for services
- Care planning of activities and services to address the agreed needs
- Coordination and referral to implement the care plan
- Regular review, monitoring and consequent adaptation of the care plan.

(Drennan and Goodman 2004, p. 527)

Hutt *et al.* (2004) note that case management may be used for a variety of reasons. Regardless of selection criteria, assessment should be a key component, with the focus varying from clinical assessment, controlling access to services, and provision and coordination of different services. They further state that although the focus of nurse-led case management is on clinical needs, minimising symptoms and reducing hospitalisation, nurse case managers play a key role in coordinating services from other health and social care providers. The overall aim of case management is to provide a holistic health and social package of care to meet the needs of the most vulnerable patients with the most complex conditions, who have often not previously been actively managed by the whole care system.

DISEASE-SPECIFIC CARE MANAGEMENT

The intention of the NSFs has been to provide a structured evidence-based framework for all health care professionals and organisations to ensure equity of care and responsive specialist services for people with LTCs. NSFs have tended to concentrate on condition-specific areas, although broader NSFs, such as those for older people and children, look at the specific needs of groups, rather than at conditions. For people with more unstable LTCs who do not necessarily require a case management approach but do require more frequent intervention or specialist support, evidence-based guidelines (Chapter 8) can assist primary health care teams in developing appropriate referral criteria and systems to ensure that this help is readily available. Specialist nurses in areas such as diabetes or epilepsy are an invaluable source of expertise to provide additional help and guidance. People needing more specialist input and support should be identified through the process of regular review (Chapter 7). Referral criteria derived from NSFs and evidence-based guidelines can then be built into an appropriate practice protocol or multi-disciplinary care pathway to ensure prompt referral and specialist support. The DoH (2005c) suggests a number of key actions to improve disease-specific care management. These are listed in Table 3.2.

Table 3.2 Key actions to improve disease-specific care management

---

- Examination of current delivery of disease management;
- establishment of multi-disciplinary professional teams with specialist support to manage care across all settings;
- identification and pro-active management of those with LTCs, using agreed standards and protocols;
- use of prompts and reminders (such as text messaging) to recall patients;
- regular review and support of those with LTCs;
- use of National Service Frameworks and quality indicators to provide a detailed approach to care.

(adapted from DoH 2005c)

PAUSE FOR REFLECTION

How do you differentiate between those needing disease-specific care management and those requiring case management?

ROLE OF THE DISTRICT NURSE IN THE MANAGEMENT OF PEOPLE WITH LTCS

Department of Health policies set out a clear strategy to develop sustainable, inclusive and equal health care for every individual to access a suitable health professional based on individual need (DoH 2004b). The publication of the NSF for long-term conditions (DoH 2005d) (although built upon the specific needs of those with long-term neurological LTCs, it is applicable to all those with LTCs) further strengthens the need for person-centred care and collaborative approaches between health and social care to ensure people can be supported at home. Indeed, Wilson (2005) noted that a number of the eleven quality requirements set out in the NSF are extremely pertinent to district nursing. These include:

- provision of a person-centred service through integrated assessment and care planning and provision of information, education, advice and support (QR1);
- community rehabilitation and support, emphasising that rehabilitation in the home is cost-effective, reduces restrictions related to daily living and improves individual well-being (QR5);
- providing personal care and support, with people able to exercise choice over where they wish to live (QR8);
- palliative care, a role well established by district nurses (QR9).

The NSF for older people (WAG 2006b) identified that social health and care needs, including for those with LTCs, should be managed effectively within the community in order to avoid inappropriate admissions to hospital. This requires holistic assessment to ensure prompt identification of problems, which district nurses undertake on a daily basis within their role.

District nurses, as members of the PHCT, deliver care in a range of settings and are well placed to deliver health education, health promotion, holistic assessment and management of people with LTCs. The advantages for patients are flexible services to meet their individual needs, ensuring continuity of care with the opportunity to be supported within the home. A study undertaken by Litaker and Moin (2003) demonstrated that patients with LTCs experience fewer exacerbations of their conditions, and consequently fewer hospital admissions, if district nurses manage their care. Historically district nurses have always managed patients with LTCs; however, this has often been in an ad hoc manner, rather than the structured case management approach advocated by the community matron/APN role. Wilson (2005) notes that district nurses were probably most enabled to deliver the holistic approach suggested by today's policies prior to the imposition of the clear boundaries between health and social care needs formed in the early 1990s.

The main focus of the district nurse has been caring for people who are housebound. Many of these people, who are often elderly, have significant co-morbidities or have been diagnosed with more than one LTC. Coordinating the care for this group of patients supports the case management model of care (DoH 2007), the difference being that for these patients their preliminary contact with the district nursing service may be for an unrelated problem and it is only during the initial assessment process that problems are identified. Community matrons are expected to actively seek out people who would benefit from a case management approach using appropriate data. *First Assessment* (Audit Commission 1999) concluded that one of the skills that district nurses consistently demonstrated was their ability to conduct holistic assessments, which is essential in order to manage patients with LTCs. Effective assessment ensures that the patient is provided with evidence-based care and it is an essential requirement of all members of the district nursing team. Older people often have complex needs that change rapidly. To ensure their safe management within the home environment requires the development and delivery of individual care plans. District nurses use a broad approach towards assessment, reassessing patients at each visit, acknowledging their changing needs and referring to other health care professionals where necessary. Advanced health assessment skills are also among the main requirements for the community matron role, along with expert clinical skills, the key difference appearing to be in the advanced educational preparation recommended to carry out the community matron role.

The introduction of the new General Medical Services (nGMS) contract (BMA/NHS Confederation 2003) has enabled district nurses working within the

PHCT to have a clearer focus when providing care to this sometimes vulnerable group of patients. Providing annual reviews for patients within their own homes is now commonplace, ensuring a more equitable health care service. Research supports the view that hospital admissions are prevented by the intervention of a district nurse (Bernabei *et al.* 1998; Gagnon 1999). It can be established that care is less fragmented as district nurses are able to signpost patients to the most appropriate services. The DoH (2006a) discusses the importance of supporting and caring for people in their home environment, rather than in secondary care, particularly those over age 65 and those with an LTC. It also stresses the need to work more closely with social services to support this group of people to allow them to remain at home. Of all the PHCT, the district nurse will have key working knowledge of the social service network within the local area of practice and would therefore seem to be the person most able to organise care. It is often the most 'sick' patients who are visited by the district nurse when an exacerbation of their condition makes it impossible for them to attend the GP surgery.

It would be fair to conclude that although recognised as experts in case management of highly complex patients with LTCs, district nurses run the risk of losing out on this element of their role if they fail to be responsive to policy initiatives. There are new roles being developed which will certainly cross over with the district nurses' position and may well leave them mopping up the problems from other services (Bennett and Robinson 2005). Recent years have seen health policies developed, which although not directed at district nursing services have undoubtedly had a huge impact on their work and how they deliver care. District nurses are faced with a challenge of self-perception; they should now see themselves as impressively adapted to professional and organisational change and politically influential, as the policy spotlight is clearly on improved and systematic management of LTCs.

ROLE OF THE PRACTICE NURSE IN THE MANAGEMENT OF PEOPLE WITH LTCS

In the UK the DoH (1990) GP contract laid the foundations for moving primary care services away from a curative, illness-led service to that of a preventive health promotion-led service. GPs, through a system of financial reimbursement, were encouraged to promote health as well as treat illness, by providing services such as well person health checks and chronic disease management clinics. In order to provide these services GPs employed more practice nurses (PNs).

The rise of the clinical governance agenda (DoH 1998) put an increasing emphasis not only on the provision of evidence-based care, but also on procedures such as audits in order to monitor both the quality of the care provided to patients and the quality of the organisational set-up providing this care. In the primary care setting practice nurses took on much of the responsibility for providing this quality care, developing their skills and knowledge accordingly. As a profession, general practice nursing evolved rapidly, with numbers across the UK increasing from 3,500 in 1990 to 24,959 in 2003 (RCGP 2004). The importance of strategic and systematic care of patients with LTCs, which began with the 1990 GP contract, including the 3 Rs – registration, regular recall and review (DoH 2005c) – was further emphasised with the publication of NSFs, the first of which to be introduced in the UK was the *NSF for Coronary Heart Disease* (DoH 2000a). Practice nurses quickly rose to the challenge of providing this care. By this time they had clearly demonstrated their ability to deliver effective management and strategies for people with LTCs, specifically in relation to asthma, chronic obstructive pulmonary disease (COPD), diabetes, hypertension and coronary heart disease. The nGMS (BMA/NHS Confederation 2003), implemented in 2004, created a further expansion of the role with practice nurses progressively taking on the responsibility of meeting the demands of the QOF outlined in Chapter 1.

The role of the practice nurse in regard to caring for those with LTCs includes identification, diagnosis, monitoring and management in the primary care environment:

- Identify patients for screening.
- Undertake diagnostic tests, for example spirometry.
- Contribute to the updating of long-term condition registers through accurate record keeping.
- Work within evidence-based practice protocols to provide programmes of care including annual review, initial and ongoing education and preventive advice.
- Review medication, assess adherence and develop concordance.
- Prescribe medication as appropriate (having undertaken a recognised prescribing qualification).
- Provide support and advice for patients and their carers.
- Provide advice relating to voluntary, community and patient organisations (e.g. Diabetes UK) as appropriate.
- Refer to local educational programmes such as Expert.
- Refer to other health and social care professionals as necessary.

PNs therefore play a significant role the management of people with LTCs in relation to both disease-specific care management and in supporting people to self-care. It is not just in the UK that PNs are seen as key providers in caring for patients with long-term conditions. Although the US health care system has not adopted the role, in other countries such as parts of Europe and New Zealand PNs carry out a similar role to that in the UK. In Australia PNs have not yet been identified as key stakeholders in the coordinated care service delivery model (Patterson *et al.* 2007).

ROLE OF THE MULTI-DISCIPLINARY TEAM IN THE MANAGEMENT OF PEOPLE WITH LTCS

In addition to receiving care from those in other identified nursing roles, people with LTCs may be seen by many health and social care professionals, with multi-disciplinary teams playing a key part in managing care across settings (DoH 2005c). In order for disease-specific care management to be effective, people with LTCs need to be able to access multi-professional teams based in primary or community care who can provide them with specialist advice tailored to individual need (DoH 2005c). The Royal Pharmaceutical Society of Great Britain and the British Medical Association (BMA) (2000) produced a report on teamworking in primary care. The review of the research demonstrated that benefits of teamwork could be classified as: a more responsive and patient-centred service and a more clinically and/or cost-effective service which provided more satisfying team roles and career paths for health care professionals. Their recommendations in relation to teams and team members are summarised in Table 3.3.

Table 3.3 Teams and team members

The team should:

- recognise and include the patient, carer or representative as an essential member of the primary health care team;
- establish a common, agreed purpose;
- agree set objectives and monitor progress towards them; involve all team members in decision-making and delivery of agreed objectives;
- agree team working conditions, including process for resolving conflict;
- ensure each team member understands and acknowledges the skills and knowledge of others;
- pay particular attention to communication, using technology to assist;
- ensure the practice population understands and accepts the way the team works;
- select the leader for his or her leadership skills, not by hierarchy, status or availability; include all relevant professions in the team;
- promote teamwork across health and social care;
- evaluate teamworking initiatives and develop practice based on sound evidence;
- ensure sharing of patient information is in accordance with legal and professional requirements.

(adapted from Royal Pharmaceutical Society/BMA 2000, p. 7)

Examples of effective multi-disciplinary teams

A number of systematic reviews and research studies have evaluated the use of multi-disciplinary teams in contributing to the care of people with LTCs. These include a review by McAlister *et al.* (2004), which concluded that multi-disciplinary teams were cost-effective and reduced hospital admission and overall mortality in patients with heart failure. Jackson *et al.* (2005) reviewed the care of over 82,000 patients with diabetes in 177 clinics and noted that weekly multi-disciplinary team meetings, special teams or protocols for clinical issues were among a list of factors that contributed to improved glycaemic control. The Leeds Young Adult Team provides multi-disciplinary input (physiotherapy, occupational therapy, speech and language therapy and psychology with access to contraceptive and sexual health services, social workers and consultants in rehabilitation medicine) to young adults (aged 16–25 years) with a physical impairment. The team focuses on each individual's needs and provides information, support and treatment to enable each young person to live the kind of life they choose to lead. A retrospective cohort study of the effectiveness of this approach to care found that it produced better results at no extra cost compared to an ad hoc approach (Bent *et al.* 2000). The DoH (2005c) outlines a number of examples where collaborative working has enhanced patient care. One example provided is that of a help desk set up in an ambulance dispatch centre to alert GPs to patients who have contacted the service regarding exacerbation of their condition, but who were not admitted to hospital. This ensures that the GP can closely monitor those patients and avoid potential emergency admissions in the future.

In order for a multi-disciplinary team to be effective, roles and boundaries need to be apparent, with each team member aware of his or her role and the role of others. Boundaries can sometimes be blurred, so transparent referral criteria need to be established, with clear channels of communication open to all team members. Protocols can provide an effective way of defining the role of each team member, preventing both omissions and duplication of care. Service users should also have the opportunity to be involved in discussions and decisions made about their care. A multi-disciplinary team involved in the care of a patient with diabetes may include:

- practice nurse and/or diabetes specialist nurse
- district nurse
- diabetologist and/or GP
- dietician
- podiatrist
- optician/ophthalmologist
- pharmacist
- consultant from other medical specialty (e.g. renal, cardiology, vascular).

In order that the patient/client receives optimal care all decisions should be communicated to those involved in the care. Advances in information technology, with instant access to results and patient records for all members of the team, can enhance the care provided. Specialist nurses can often provide the expertise and support that a patient requires, liaising with appropriate services and advising patients on suitable options. Multi-disciplinary teams can both contribute to and improve the pro-active care provided to patients/clients with LTCs. Evidence-based care pathways and local protocols should guide health and social care professionals in delivering appropriate packages of care.

CONCLUSION

Providing appropriate care for people with LTCs, particularly at levels 2 and 3, case management and disease-specific care management (DoH 2005c; NHPAC 2006) can be complex and often involves a number of different health and social care professionals. Whatever type of approach or model of care is adopted, the key to successful management includes regular and systematic review, adequate communication and referral criteria between all team members, including the patient/client and carer, and appropriate systems in place to support patients/clients both in times of stability and during exacerbations.

KEY POINTS

- The majority of patients with LTCs are able to self-care but adequate systems need to be put into place to provide case management and disease-specific care management programmes for those patients/clients with more complex needs.
- Where case management is adopted identification of appropriate patients is paramount and clear guidelines need to be set.
- The importance of existing nursing roles such as district nursing and practice nursing should be acknowledged and they should be provided with adequate resources and training.
- Multi-disciplinary teams should utilise evidence-based care pathways and protocols to maximise care.

FURTHER AREAS TO CONSIDER

- Are there any good examples in your area relating to multi-disciplinary teamworking?
- How does your team ensure that you communicate effectively to maximise patient care and avoid omission/duplication of services?
- How do you identify people with more complex needs who may benefit from case management?

CHAPTER 4

IMPORTANCE OF SELF-MANAGEMENT

OVERVIEW

What do we mean by self-care and what implications does this approach have on the patient–practitioner relationship? How do practitioners determine who is suitable for self-care? An overview of research studies relating to the encouragement of self-care is provided, as is a guide to how these can be implemented in the practical setting. The concept behind the expert patient is discussed, alongside the concept of developing the nurse/ client relationship to move away from the traditional paradigm of reliance on health care providers and towards a self-care/self-management para- digm, including the development of concordance and involvement of family and carers. This chapter also includes a guide to currently available schemes such as the UK's Expert Patients Programme (EPP).

INTRODUCTION AND DEFINITION

The terms 'self-care/self-management' have become progressively more popular as both the incidence of chronic/long-term conditions and the subsequent demand on health care providers increase. In part this is also due to the move away from the traditional 'medical' model of care with its focus on disease and cure and the realisation that responsibility for health lies with both society and the individual. Instead of focusing purely on curative techniques and treatments, health care providers are increasingly appreciating the value of empowering patients/clients with the skills and knowledge to manage their own condition, adapting treatment and management to fit in with individual lifestyles. The new models of care indicate a shift for chronically ill patients away from being passive recipients of care towards being partners with health professionals in managing their own care (Holman and Lorig 2000). Barlow *et al.* (2002) define self-management as 'the ability of the patient to deal with all that a chronic illness entails, including symptoms, treatment, physical and social consequences, and lifestyle changes'.

Self-management is applicable not only to those with physical long-term conditions but also to those experiencing mental health problems. The Rethink *Self-management* project (2006) defines self-management as being about 'taking control of your life and being active in your own recovery'. They further state that 'a decision to self-manage can be a key factor contributing to a person's recovery'.

Self-management for Long-term Conditions, a King's Fund publication (Corben and Rosen 2005), emphasises that although up to a quarter of those affected with long-tem conditions have more severe symptoms, the majority lead full and active lives, providing much of their care themselves, these decisions and behaviours constituting 'self-management'. Indeed, a quote from the National Service Framework (NSF) for Diabetes (DoH 2002) sums the message up succinctly: 'On average a patient with diabetes spends 3 hours per year with a health professional and the remaining 8757 hours left to manage his/her own condition.'

The World Health Organisation's (2002b) *Framework for Innovative Care of Chronic Conditions* identifies self-management support as one of the building blocks for effective health care organisations, stating that health care workers are crucial in educating patients and families about self-management and that health care workers must support patients' self-management efforts over time. Recent government policy in countries such as the USA, Canada, Australia, New Zealand, Asia and here in the UK has increasingly focused on promoting self-care strategies and identifying appropriate support for enabling self-care. Initiatives such as Stanford University's *Chronic Disease Self-management Programme* (Lorig *et al.* 1999), the UK's *Expert Patient Programme* and Australia's *Sharing Health Care Initiative* (Australian Government Department of Health and Ageing 2007) set the scene for the way forward in health care provision for those with long-term condition(s). The key to these programmes is to provide individuals with the skills to coordinate everything needed to manage their health, as well as to help them keep active.

IS SELF-MANAGEMENT EFFECTIVE? EVIDENCE SUPPORTING SELF-MANAGEMENT INTERVENTIONS

Current policy initiatives have clearly paved the way forward for the integration of self-management strategies into chronic illness programmes. But does self-management improve overall health outcomes and what types of intervention have been shown to be effective? Wagner *et al.* (2001) suggest that self-management skills are essential and highlight the importance of including patient-oriented interventions when designing systems of care that meet the needs of the chronically ill. They observe that historically pioneers of chronic disease management have emphasised that effective management requires systems of care that are designed to help patients meet the challenges of chronic disease. Furthermore, they underline that reviews of earlier literature on chronic disease interventions noted that those that had a positive effect on patient well-being included systematic efforts to increase patients' knowledge, skills and confidence to manage their condition.

Renders *et al.* (2001) confirmed this view in a systematic review, undertaken for the Cochrane Library, which examined interventions to improve primary care for diabetes. The review identified that successful approaches tended to be the all-round interventions that included elements such as continuing education, physician feedback and patient-oriented interventions of an educational and supportive nature. They noted that interventions targeting health care providers' behaviour were unsuccessful in changing patient outcomes, unless they were accompanied by patient-directed interventions. Rees and Williams (2008) make the point that the effectiveness of self-care management may have different meanings for different practitioners and clients. To effectively partner and support patients with self-care management, an understanding and recognition of patient knowledge and expertise is vital.

The notion of patient-centred care and self-management has its critics, however, with Robb and Seddon (2006) surmising that questions have been raised both about the extent to which a patient may be considered an 'expert' and also about the implications for healthcare practitioners in accepting patients taking a more active role in their care. They suggest that these arguments can largely be addressed through distinguishing between 'illness' and 'disease', suggesting that 'illness' is something experienced uniquely by the individual in terms of symptoms and how he or she manages and experiences the condition. On the other hand, 'disease' is something understood and managed by health care professionals and requires technical expertise based on knowledge of the condition, appropriate treatment and uncertain presentations. The key, they conclude, is in developing effective collaborative partnerships between patients/clients and practitioners.

Examples of patient-directed interventions

Problem-solving skills

Bodenheimer *et al.* (2002, p. 2469) emphasise that whereas traditional patient education offers information and technical skills, self-management education teaches problem-solving skills. Their review of evidence from controlled clinical trials suggests that:

1   Programmes teaching self-management skills are more effective than information-only patient education in improving clinical outcomes.
2   In some circumstances, self-management education improves outcomes and can reduce costs for arthritis and probably for adult asthma patients.
3   In initial studies, a self-management education programme bringing together patients with a variety of chronic conditions may improve outcomes and reduce costs.

A systematic review of the literature on problem-solving and its associations with diabetes self-management and control (Hill-Briggs and Gemmell 2007) concluded that cross-sectional studies in adults, but not in children/ adolescents, provided consistent evidence of associations between problem-solving and HbA1c level (a key indicator of glycaemic control in diabetes). They defined problem-solving as 'a multidimensional construct encompassing verbal reasoning/rational problem solving, quantitative problem solving, and coping'. Despite methodological limitations 25 per cent of problem-solving intervention studies with children/adolescents and 50 per cent of interventions with adults reported improvement in HbA1c. Most intervention studies reported an improvement in behaviour, most commonly global adherence in children/ adolescents and dietary behaviour in adults.

Action plans

Handley *et al.* (2006) define an action plan as 'an agreement between clinician and patient that the patient will make a specific behaviour change'. Handley *et al.*'s (2006) descriptive study based in a primary care setting involved 228 patients across eight primary care sites. Fifty-three per cent of patients reported making a behaviour change based on the action plan, suggesting that action plans may be a useful strategy to encourage behaviour change for patients seen in primary care.

Action plans have been noted as successful in assisting patients in self-management of specific conditions, asthma in particular. A systematic review by

Powell and Gibson (2002) concluded that optimisation of asthma control by self-adjustment of medications with the aid of a written action plan was equivalent to that by regular medical review. Individualised written action plans based on PEF (peak expiratory flow) measurements were equivalent to action plans based on symptoms. Toelle and Ram (2004) in a later review, however, suggested that there is not enough evidence to show that personalised, written self-management plans for asthma, as the sole intervention, improve health outcomes. They conclude that to change asthma management behaviour and improve health outcomes requires a coordinated approach of self-management education, regular review and a written action plan.

In other conditions, for example COPD (chronic obstructive pulmonary disease), the effectiveness of action plans is unknown. Turnock et al.'s (2005) systematic review concludes that although there is evidence that action plans help people with COPD to recognise and react appropriately to an exacerbation of their symptoms via the self-initiation of antibiotics or steroids, there was no evidence of significant effects on health care utilisation, health-related quality of life, lung function, functional capacity, symptom scores, mortality, anxiety or depression.

Self-management education

A particular focus of governmental policy is on encouraging patients to become 'experts' in their own conditions. Recent systematic reviews have begun to examine the effectiveness of these interventions in relation to different long-term conditions. A systematic review by Foster et al. (2007) reviewed the efficacy of lay-led self-management programmes for a range of chronic conditions, including arthritis, diabetes, hypertension and chronic pain. The results suggested small, short-term improvements in participants' self-efficacy, self-rated health, cognitive symptom management and frequency of aerobic exercise, but there was no evidence that they improved psychological health, symptoms or health-related quality of life, or that they significantly altered health care use. Riemsa et al. (2003), in reviewing patient education programmes in relation to rheumatoid arthritis, indicated significant short-term benefits related to disability, joint counts, patient global assessment, psychological status, and depression and pain. However, at long-term follow-up no significant effects of patient education were found.

Stokes et al. (2007) reviewed the evidence relating to self-management in epilepsy in children and young people. Only one trial met their criteria for inclusion in the review, and this study suggested that self-management education may reduce the number of seizures and improve other aspects of people's lives such as fear of and knowledge about epilepsy, but the quality of the trial meant no recommendations could be made regarding the overall effectiveness of the programme or what it should consist of. A similar picture was seen in the review undertaken by Effing *et al.* (2007) in relation to self-management education in patients with COPD. Due to the wide variations in the studies relating to interventions, study populations and follow-up periods, no clear recommendations could be made, although Effing *et al.* (2007) concluded that it was likely that self-management education is associated with a reduction in hospital admissions with no indications of detrimental effects in other outcome parameters.

Van Dam *et al.*'s (2003) systematic review approached patient education from a different viewpoint. They focused on reviewing studies that educated and empowered patients to participate in care (relating to diabetes) in addition, or in comparison, to altering health care provider behaviour. They concluded that supporting patients to participate in care and self-behaviour (through interventions such as assistant-guided patient preparation for visits to doctors, empowering group education, group consultations) was effective in engaging patients with diabetes in self-care management and positively affecting self-care outcomes, and was more effective than focusing on health care provider behaviour. This demonstrates that education should not simply focus on individual conditions but should aim to empower individuals to take responsibility for their health care provision to ensure that their needs are being met.

Patient–practitioner encounter

Rees and Williams (2008) reviewed the patient–practitioner encounter in relation to adults living in the community with chronic illness. They considered all rigorous quantitative and qualitative studies where self-care was the focus including the review undertaken by Renders *et al.* (2001) mentioned earlier. Professional interventions such as education, and organisational interventions such as management of regular review and follow up, were shown to improve process outcomes in the management of a patient–practitioner encounter. However, the addition of patient-oriented interventions, such as patient education and/or enhanced nursing involvement, led to improved health outcomes. Interventions shown to be effective were: information-giving, including the use of a guidebook, the use of care plans, the structure of treatment using checklists, and education and support for staff in 'collaboratives' (p. 2).

Nurses in particular were shown to have an effective role in educating patients and facilitating adherence to treatment, with patients finding nurses approachable. Patients were more likely to contact a nurse regarding their care when given the opportunity. Organisational factors such as time, resources and the opportunity to have 'open access' to appointments were also found to have an impact, as well as comprehensive and user-friendly information to enhance communication between patients and practitioners. Overall, Rees and Williams (2008) concluded that patient-focused interventions do have a positive effect on patient self-care outcomes. They emphasise that when assessing the effectiveness of interventions aimed at improving self-care outcomes the focus should not solely be on measurement of medical indicators but should accept and value patients' experiences of self-care management and reflect the patients' cultural view. They recommend that further qualitative research studies regarding patients' self-care and health outcomes and behaviours are needed to establish which are the most effective patient-focused interventions.

PAUSE FOR REFLECTION

What strategies do you use to encourage patients to self-manage? How do you determine if these are effective?

STRATEGIES FOR SUCCESSFUL SELF-MANAGEMENT

Chronic conditions vary considerably in numerous ways: signs and symptoms – both physical and mental – rate of progression, degree of disability and short- and long-term outcomes to name but a few. Successful self-management, however, involves development of a number of key skills, as in all chronic conditions. These are listed in Table 4.1.

Corbin and Rosen's (2005) King's Fund working paper, reviewing literature on patients' perspectives about self-management, identified that people diagnosed with a long-term condition must make a series of adjustments to their lives and also recognised that individuals respond differently over time. They identified three themes that shaped people's responses to self-management:

- The different ways in which people receive their diagnosis
- The fact that different people have different responses
- The fact that people's ability to self-manage changes over time.

(Corbin and Rosen 2005, p. 3)

Table 4.1 Key skills for successful self-management

- Knowledge of the condition;
- how to manage symptoms;
- ability to manage medication (including evaluating new treatments);
- how to respond to changes in condition;
- awareness of deterioration;
- when to seek medical help;
- how to work effectively with your health care team;
- awareness of how your lifestyle choices can affect your condition.

In order for service providers to support self-management effectively Corbin and Rosen (2005, p. 7) identified three more key themes:

- The importance of good relationships between professionals and patients
- The need for patients to have clear information about their condition and guidance on how to access it
- The need for flexibility in service provision to fit in with patients' other commitments.

The review clearly emphasised the importance of a good relationship between professional and patient to support self-management and identified a number of important aspects that need to be in place that will enhance the patient–professional encounter (Table 4.2).

They also acknowledge that not everyone will want or be able to self-manage. They emphasise that some patients will always prefer their management to be health care provider (physician or nurse) led, whereas for others the nature and amount of their involvement will alter at different stages of their condition. Factors influencing active self-management may include time since diagnosis, disease severity, age, social support and level of education, with those who lack basic literacy skills possibly less likely to self-manage well (Corbin and Rosen 2005).

Rees and Williams (2008) propose that patient-oriented interventions are the most effective in achieving good self-care behavioural and health outcomes, with patient participation in the patient–practitioner encounter a key factor. They suggest some key implications for practice in relation to self-management (Table 4.3).

In addition, they suggest that professionals need to recognise and value patients' views and experiences in order to support their self-care management, which, as they appreciate, involves social as well as medical management. Consultations should: avoid being medically focused; aim to share knowledge and information; endorse the patient's view that he or she is the most reliable and accurate source of information about his or her physiological function; trust the patients' interpretations of their physiological function, and modify advice in response to patients in accordance with their bodily cues and experiences (Rees and Williams 2008).

Table 4.2 Aspects that will enhance the patient–professional encounter

---

The ability to:

- Listen
- Identify the patient's main concerns
- Allow time for discussion
- Understand how the patient experiences their condition
- Ensure that the patient contributes to the planning of their care.

(Corbin and Rosen 2005, p. 7)

Table 4.3 Implications for practice

- Provide clear concise information at diagnosis and from then onwards
- Enable and encourage patient participation during the patient–practitioner encounter
- Provide opportunities for patients to talk about their diet, routines and lifestyle management within the encounter
- Build in extra time in consultations
- Utilise care plans and self-management plans to help facilitate discussion
- Share medical and nursing knowledge, and recognise the value of patients' knowledge and experiences
- Ensure nurse involvement, as nurses relate well to patients who want to discuss self-care management.

(Rees and Williams 2008, p. 3)

WHO'S SUITABLE FOR SELF-CARE?

Numerous reviews and research studies have attempted to determine which patients/clients may be better able to self-manage. When assessing patients it is important that all the factors influencing their current state of health are taken into account and that a holistic approach is taken to care, including reviewing physical, psychological and social need. Some of the potential factors that may influence an individual's ability to self-care have been indicated earlier such as age, disease severity and social support, but it is important to remember that health and social needs change over time. This is particularly relevant for those with long-term conditions and patients should continue to be provided with the opportunity to self-manage throughout their lifetime. Individuals who prefer their care to be health professional led should not be disadvantaged and should continue to receive the same high level of care as those who choose to take a more interactive role.

DEVELOPING CONCORDANCE/EMPOWERMENT/ SHARED DECISION-MAKING/PATIENT-CENTRED CARE

Issues surrounding behaviour change strategies will be discussed in the next chapter but it is important at this stage to note some of the key terms used when developing the nurse/client relationship to move away from the traditional paradigm of reliance on health care providers and towards a self-care/self-management paradigm. Shared decision-making is a term that is very much on today's agenda, in relation not only to long-term conditions but also to those presenting with more acute self-limiting illnesses. Suffice to say that patient- or person-centred care should involve provision of systems that are patient- rather than service-led, involve individuals in making decisions about their ongoing health care choices, respect those decisions, provide effective treatment, emotional support and empathy, involve families and carers and ensure continuity of care wherever possible. Concordance rather than compliance should be the key to all patient–provider interactions, informing individuals about the most effective treatment options and ensuring that they understand all the options available, including the pros and cons of choosing or rejecting a plan of care, but respecting their decisions as to how they interpret and apply those treatment options.

SELF-MANAGEMENT PROGRAMMES

The Chronic Disease Self-management Programme

Stanford University's Chronic Disease Self-management Programme developed by Kate Lorig (see Lorig *et al.* 1999) began initially in the 1970s at the Stanford Patient Education Research Center, California, USA, originally focusing on self-help skills for people living with arthritis. The theoretical underpinning of the concept is 'self-efficacy', which was developed as a concept by Albert Bandura, a Canadian psychologist, also based at Stanford. The initial Arthritis Self-help Course, which is now offered worldwide, became the model for a number of other programmes such as the Chronic Disease Self-management Programme, the Positive Self-management Programme for HIV/AIDS and the Back Pain Self-management Programme to name but a few.

The Center develops and delivers community-based self-management programmes to improve the physical and emotional health of participants living with chronic illness while reducing health care costs, with their main mission being research. All the programmes offered by the Center undergo a rigorous two- to four-year evaluation before being released for wider dissemination. A number of internet versions of the programmes are currently under evaluation, further details of which may be found at: http://patienteducation.stanford.edu/programs/.

The Chronic Disease Self-management Programme covers the following key areas:

1 Techniques to deal with problems such as frustration, fatigue, pain and isolation.
2 Appropriate exercise for maintaining and improving strength, flexibility and endurance.
3 Appropriate use of medications.
4 Communicating effectively with family, friends and health professionals.
5 Nutrition.
6 How to evaluate new treatments.
   (http://patienteducation.stanford.edu/programs/cdsmp.html)

The Chronic Disease Self-management Programme has three distinct features: it was developed using the experiences of people living with long-term conditions as a starting point; it is run in community settings, and it is lay-led by pairs of trained leaders who themselves have a long-term condition. The programme has since been adopted worldwide (as the EPP in the UK, the Chronic Disease Self-management Programme in British Columbia, Canada, and other adaptations in Europe, Asia, Australia and New Zealand), the key to its success being the way in which it is taught: highly participative classes which encourage mutual support and success to build the participants' confidence in their ability to manage their health and maintain active and fulfilling lives. Programmes are run as interactive workshops over a period of time (generally two hours a week over a six-week period), where people with different chronic diseases attend together. It teaches the skills needed in the day-to-day management of treatment and to maintain and/or increase life's activities.

The Expert Patients Programme (UK)

In the UK the Living with Long-term Illness (LILL) Project was set up in September 1998 to increase knowledge about, and use of, self-management programmes for people living with long-term conditions. The overall aims included the creation of a self-management information-sharing network, the facilitation of robust monitoring and evaluation processes and the mapping of existing self-management interventions (DoH 2006b).

The report from this programme fed into the Expert Patients Task Force, set up in 1999 to design a programme that would bring together the valuable work of patient and clinical organisations in developing self-management initiatives. The Department of Health (DoH 2001) followed this up with a report, *The Expert Patient: A New Approach to Chronic Disease Management for the 21st Century*, which was to lay the foundations for the EPP. Since then the programme, a lay-led self-management programme specifically for people living with long-term conditions, has grown from strength to strength. In England the EPP currently offers around 12,000 course places a year. Evaluation of the programme indicates that self-management can lead to decreased severity of symptoms and decrease in pain, as well as overall improved life satisfaction and sense of control, accompanied by increased activity levels. Some reduction in consultations with health care professionals such as GPs, consultant and accident and emergency (A&E) attendance was also noted. Full details of the evaluation may be obtained from http://www.dh.gov.uk/en/Aboutus/Ministers andDepartmentLeaders/ChiefMedicalOfficer/ProgressOnPolicy/ProgressBrowsa bleDocument/DH_4102757.

As well as the initial EPP a number of other courses have been developed for groups and communities considered marginalised. These include ethnic minority communities, with courses available in a variety of different languages, and courses specifically aimed at groups such as young people living with long-term conditions; there are also programmes designed for carers.

The EPP has also been rolled out across Wales, where it began in 2002. Each session looks at:

- Managing symptoms such as pain and tiredness
- Dealing with anger, fear and frustration
- Coping with stress, depression and low self-image
- Eating healthily
- Learning relaxation techniques and taking regular exercise
- Improved communication with family, friends and health professionals
- Planning for the future.

(Expert Patients Programme Wales 2008)

In addition to the orginal EPP a number of other courses are now also available:

- Looking After Me (a course for carers)
- In Working Condition (workshops for people who want to work)
- Dealing with Feelings (workshops for people with mild to moderate depression, stress and anxiety).

(Expert Patients Programme Wales 2008)

The overall aim of the EPP is not to review specific individual health needs or provide health condition or treatment information but to encourage people living with long-term conditions to share their skills and experience and to develop the confidence to take responsibility for their own care and to work in equal partnership with health and social care professionals (Expert Patients Programme Wales 2008).

Other educational programmes

Although the EPP is the most well-known programme and many others have evolved from the initial Chronic Disease Self-management Programme it is worth noting that there are many other programmes, often specific to particular conditions, that aim to provide individuals with the knowledge and skills with which to manage their own conditions. These include: DAFNE (Dose Adjustment for Normal Eating); DESMOND (Diabetes Education and Self Management for Ongoing and Newly Diagnosed Diabetes); Challenge Arthritis; Self Management for IBS (Irritable Bowel Syndrome), to name but a few. It is worthwhile determining what is available in your area.

ORGANISATIONS THAT ADVISE ON SELF-MANAGEMENT

A number of charitable organisations provide help and advice to support those suffering from long-term conditions and some UK examples of these are provided below with the website addresses.

Arthritis Care: Ways to Self-manage

http://www.arthritiscare.org.uk/LivingwithArthritis/Self-management/Waysto self-manage

Table 4.4 Arthritis Care: Ways to Self-manage

Self-management is about using your own resources to help manage the condition. There is much you can do for yourself. Indeed, you may well already use a combination of the following techniques:

- Keeping active will help keep your muscles strong and joints moving.
- Looking after your joints by reducing the stress on them.
- Pacing yourself – try to balance rest with activity.
- Having a warm bath and using heated pads or a hot water bottle to reduce stiffness.
- Using a cold pack or a damp cloth around ice cubes or frozen vegetables to reduce swelling.
- Complementary therapies such as homeopathy, acupuncture and osteopathy.
- Massage to help relax muscles and improve blood flow.
- Tens (Transcutaneous Electrical Nerve Stimulation) machines use electrical impulses to block pain.
- Relaxation, breathing exercises and meditation techniques to relax muscles and ease pain.

(Arthritis Care 2008)

Diabetes UK: Your Responsibilities

http://www.diabetes.org.uk/Guide-to-diabetes/What_care_to_expect/Your_ responsibilities/

Table 4.5 Diabetes UK: Your Responsibilities

It is your responsibility:

- To take as much control of your diabetes on a day-to-day basis as you can. The more you know about your own diabetes, the easier this will become.
- To learn about and practise self-care, which should include dietary education, exercise and monitoring blood glucose levels.
- To examine your feet regularly or have someone check them.
- To know how to manage your diabetes and when to ask for help if you are ill (e.g. chest infection, flu or diarrhoea and vomiting).
- To know when, where and how to contact your diabetes care team.
- To build the diabetes advice discussed with you into your daily life.
- To talk regularly with your diabetes care team and ask questions you may have.
- To make a list of points to raise at appointments, if you find it helpful.
- To attend your scheduled appointments and inform the diabetes care team if you are unable to do so.

(Diabetes UK 2006)

Asthma UK: Be in Control

http://www.asthma.org.uk/all_about_asthma/controlling_your_asthma/resources
_to_help_you/index.html.

Table 4.6 Asthma UK: Be in Control

Asthma UK's Be in Control materials have been created to help control your asthma symptoms.
The 'Be in Control' pack includes:

- Personal Asthma Action Plan – contains the information you need to keep your asthma well
  controlled; it gives you guidance about what action to take when your asthma symptoms change.
- Your Peak Flow Diary – this is for you to record your peak flow scores, alongside any symptoms
  you may be having and the medicines you are taking. It will help you recognise when your
  asthma is getting worse.
- Asthma Medicine Card – a written record of which medicines you should take and when.
- Making the Most of your Asthma Review – everyone with asthma should have an asthma review
  with their doctor or asthma nurse at least once a year. This leaflet gives you the information about
  what you should discuss at your asthma review.

(Asthma UK Cymru 2008)

Epilepsy Action: Take Control

http://www.takecontroluk.org/asp/template_aboutTakeControl.asp?id=30&sm=.

Table 4.7 Epilepsy Action: Take Control

The Epilepsy Action Take Control website provides:

- A step-by-step guide on how to make the most of Take Control.
- An easy-to-use epilepsy diary.
- Some basic information about epilepsy.

(Epilepsy Action 2008)

KEY POINTS

- The medical model of care is no longer a suitable model for those with long-term conditions.
- Self-care programmes have been in existence since the 1970s and have been subject to rigorous evaluation studies, although they are not without their critics.
- Inclusion of patient-oriented interventions has a far greater impact on health outcomes than concentrating solely on changing provider interventions.
- Not all patients/clients are suitable for self-care; all should be given the opportunity to become involved in self-management but those who choose not to should not be disadvantaged.

FURTHER AREAS TO CONSIDER

- What is the governmental policy regarding delivery of self-care programmes in your area?
- What programmes are available in your area regarding management of chronic illness/long-term conditions?
- What evaluations are taking place with regard to self-management programmes?
- What systems have been put in place in your practice area to ensure patients are provided with information relating to self-care/self-management?

CHAPTER 5

MOTIVATIONAL INTERVIEWING

Claire A. Lane

OVERVIEW

This chapter introduces simple and practical behaviour change strategies that can be initiated by clinicians to encourage self-care and motivate changes in behaviour and attitudes to health.

> We are what we repeatedly do. Excellence is, therefore, not an act, but a habit.
>
> (Aristotle)

Mr Green is 55 years old and lives with his long-term partner. Mr Green has a busy life. He works part-time doing clerical work. He also does voluntary work, regularly enjoys doing pub quizzes with his friends, and spends time with his partner, daughter and grandchildren at the weekends. He was diagnosed with this type 2 diabetes three years ago, and has still not managed to achieve good control. His body mass index (BMI) is 31. He comes in to see you once every six months or so, and every time he is disappointed to hear that his HbA1c is still at 10.2, despite the fact that he takes all his medication. It has been like this for the past two years or so.

It is easy to see where Mr Green is going wrong. To get that HbA1c down, all he needs to do is to make a few changes. He and his wife could easily eat healthier alternatives to their usual convenience food and add in a little roughage

– this wouldn't take longer to cook. If he could cut down from an average three pints of beer to two pints on a quiz night, this would make a huge difference. At the weekends, he could do some exercise-based activity with his family – for example, hiking or swimming.

The health professionals have tried telling Mr Green this. In fact, they have probably told him this a hundred times, but he just doesn't seem to make those changes. As soon as he does make those changes, things will probably be a lot better for him. If he doesn't start making those changes soon, he's looking at severe complications. Every visit, he says he will try his best to make all the changes that have been suggested. Every visit, nothing really seems to change very much. He just says he is a busy man, and he is tired a lot of the time. It's almost as if he is not taking his health seriously – besides, if he could sort out the blood sugars, this would probably make him feel a little less tired.

There are times when most of us can think of our own Mr Green: a patient who never seems to do what is best for them. Imagine that it is 3 p.m. on a Friday afternoon. You look at your list of appointments and you see that you have three patients in a row, and they are all just like Mr Green. How does this make you feel?

When asking health professionals who work with chronic disease patients this very question, many say that trying to encourage a patient like Mr Green to make health behaviour changes can be difficult, or even frustrating at times (especially at 3 p.m. on a Friday afternoon . . .). They want to make the patient better – they don't want to see his health deteriorate further.

Why is it that some patients seem to persevere and make the changes they need to make, and others do not? Why is it that sometimes we feel that we have made a difference, while at other times it just feels as though we are wading through treacle? How can we best persuade patients to make behaviour changes to help them manage their diabetes better?

This chapter aims to provide some clarity on these kinds of questions. Starting with a brief overview of theories about how and why people make changes, I will go on to describe different ways of communicating about change, and will lead on to 'motivational interviewing' (MI) (Miller and Rollnick 2002), a clinical method that practitioners can find useful when speaking to patients about behaviour change. Following some background information about how and why MI can be useful in practice, the spirit and principles of the method are illustrated, and some examples of ways in which MI can be incorporated into clinical practice are given. Finally, the evidence for MI in facilitating health behaviour change will be summarised, and some guidance given as to where you can find out more about this method of clinical practice.

UNDERSTANDING THE PROCESS OF BEHAVIOUR CHANGE

Behaviour change is something that we have all experienced. For example, think of something that you, at the present time, need to change in your life. Now ask yourself three questions:

- Do you know why you should make the change?
- Do you have a fair idea of the kinds of things you need to do to make the change?
- Have you actually made the change yet?

Some of you may have answered 'Yes' to question 3. Congratulations, and very well done! However, there are likely to be many of you who answered 'No'. What does this tell us? Mainly, it demonstrates that just because somebody knows why and how they should make a change, this in itself does not necessarily mean that they will in turn make the change. This is important to bear in mind, given that within health care contexts it is often assumed that if patients have the information about how and why to make changes, this will make them change. If they don't change, then they are given more information, and so the cycle continues. So if information deficit is not the problem, why is it that we as human beings often find it difficult to change? There are many factors that may affect how and why individuals make changes. Some of these will be discussed briefly below.

Freedom and personal autonomy

One factor that can affect our motivation to make changes is the degree to which we feel we are in control of the decision to do so. If we tell people that their personal freedom and autonomy are being taken away, that can in turn motivate them to perform the action they are told not to do (or not do what they are told). Put simply, this describes the individual who thinks 'no-one tells me what to do'. In the psychology arena, this is known as *reactance theory* (Brehm 1966).

Using our example of Mr Green, it is possible he feels that the health care professional telling him what he should do, or trying to persuade him to make changes, is taking away his sense of personal autonomy. It is important to highlight here that it is Mr Green who is in control of the changes he makes – not the clinician. Much as we would like to be able to make lifestyle changes for our patients, it is impossible for us to do so!

How you see yourself

A person's sense of identity and how they view their self can also influence their decisions regarding change. Bem (1972) argued that we develop our attitudes by observing our own behaviour and concluding what attitudes must have caused that behaviour. How individuals talk about themselves and the way in which they behave can lead them to believe that they behave in a certain way because it is the way they are.

If Mr Green can imagine not drinking three pints of beer during the pub quiz, this may in turn help him to change his existing behaviour. By the same token, if he can imagine succeeding with this change, it may also help him feel more motivated to try to change. In clinical situations, practitioners often focus on what the patient has not managed to change. Shifting focus and concentrating on the small achievements Mr Green has made may help him to alter his self-perception, which could help him to feel more able to change.

Inner conflict

When it comes to making changes, reflecting on behaviours that do not match up with our own personal beliefs can also affect our motivation to make changes. Festinger (1957) claimed that a sense of inner conflict (*cognitive dissonance*) occurs when a person behaves in a way which conflicts with their own beliefs about their self. People generally feel uncomfortable when they hold two conflicting thoughts, and this creates an urge to resolve the conflict.

For example, Mr Green may be thinking, 'I want to be healthy, but I eat a lot of food with a lot of fat and sugar in it, which is bad for me and my diabetes'. The urge to resolve this conflict could mean that he decides to gradually reduce the amount of saturated fat and sugar in his diet. However, if Mr Green does not believe he can reduce the amount of fat and sugar in his diet very easily, it may be easier to despise what he feels he cannot achieve: 'Who wants to be healthy but unhappy? Let's forget that idea.'

Ambivalence

In relation to behaviour change, the term 'ambivalence' refers to the notion of having mixed feelings, and in turn feeling unsure or indecisive. Most of us can think of a time in our lives when we have had to make a decision, and have been torn between different courses of action. This may have raised feelings of conflict about which course of action is the best, or a sense of hopelessness when neither path seems to lead to a completely satisfactory ending.

Looking at the example of Mr Green again, we can all see the 'damage' he is doing to himself through eating unhealthy foods, not taking enough exercise, and drinking a little too much alcohol. It is natural to want to stop Mr Green taking part in these harmful activities – after all, it is often the desire to help, and improve the health of others, that draws people into careers in health care in the first place.

Mr Green may feel several different ways about making those changes. He can see how changing will be beneficial to his health and quality of life. Conversely, however, he may also see that it will be hard to change. Such changes may affect other family members, and he may perceive a negative impact on their social life. He may not enjoy some of the things he has been told he should do, or feel unhappy about giving up behaviours that until now have been pleasurable. This is the essence of ambivalence about making changes to health behaviours, which often makes the decision to change a difficult one.

Readiness, importance and confidence

Another factor that may affect patients' motivation to change is their 'readiness' to make changes. One model commonly used to try to understand readiness is the 'stages of change' component of the trans-theoretical model of change (Prochaska and DiClemente 1983). This model describes five possible stages that individuals may be at in terms of making a change:

- Pre-contemplation stage – the person has not even considered that they may need to make changes at this point.
- Contemplation stage – the person has considered that there is something he or she probably needs to change.
- Preparation stage – the person makes plans as to how he or she might change.
- Action stage – the person is actively undertaking behavioural changes.
- Maintenance stage – the person maintains the changes he or she made in the action stage over a period of time.

The stages are not linear – an individual can relapse and fall back into former stages at any point in time. For example, perhaps the changes made in the action stage were difficult to implement, causing a person to fall back into the contemplation or preparation stage, or a stressful life event such as a relationship breakup forced the person back into the pre-contemplation stage for a time.

Two factors that can influence an individual's readiness to make changes are the degree of *importance* he or she attaches to making the behaviour change, and the *confidence* to achieve it (Keller and White 1997; Rollnick *et al.* 2007). Having the confidence to achieve change is recognised as a great factor in making lifestyle changes. If a person believes he or she can change this is often half the battle. If people do not believe they can change they may not even try (Bandura 1995). In general, if importance and confidence are both high, the person is more likely to feel ready to make changes. If importance and confidence are both low, they are not likely to feel at all ready to make changes. If importance and confidence are somewhere in the middle of high and low, or either importance or confidence is high but the other is low, the individual is likely to be *ambivalent* about making changes.

Bearing this in mind, if the practitioner could find out where Mr Green is in terms of his readiness to make changes, he or she could choose the most helpful style in which to talk with him about change. This concept of communication styles is discussed in more detail below.

STYLE COUNCIL

As human beings, we use different styles of communication in different situations in our everyday lives. The styles that we adopt in clinical practice with patients vary – both from patient to patient, and also from issue to issue. We may, for example, find the need to switch styles multiple times during a consultation.

Rollnick *et al.* (2007) developed a simple three-styles model for understanding how practitioners approach problem solving in everyday practice:

- directing
- following
- guiding.

A *directing* style is widely used in health and social care to solve problems. It involves provision of expert advice and help and, done skilfully, is well timed and personally relevant, while not damaging rapport with the patient.

A *following* style describes the approach whereby a clinician offers support and encouragement through carefully listening to the patient's situation. The following style is most prevalent in scenarios such as breaking bad news, or when trying to understand why a patient is upset or distressed.

Finally, a *guiding* style involves the clinician and the patient working collaboratively to help the patient identify solutions to a problem. Both practitioner and patient are active in this process. Guiding can be most effective in discussions about issues such as skill acquisition or making difficult lifestyle changes. This is where MI fits in: it has been defined *as a refined form of guiding* (Rollnick *et al.* 2007).

Skilful communication in practice involves switching flexibly between these styles according to the patient's needs. When it comes to talking about health behaviour changes with ambivalent patients, the guiding style is likely to be the most effective.

So what is MI, and how does it fit in with a guiding style? This is discussed in more detail in the next section.

MOTIVATIONAL INTERVIEWING

Motivational interviewing is defined as 'a client-centered, directive style for enhancing intrinsic motivation to change by exploring and resolving ambivalence' (Miller and Rollnick 2002). It has traditionally been practised within the addictions field and other specialist, help-seeking clinical settings, with consultation times ranging from approximately 30 minutes to an hour in length. In recent times, however, MI has been adapted for use in much briefer consultations in a range of other environments, including general health care settings (Rollnick *et al.* 1999, 2007).

As we have seen above, ambivalence can be a barrier to making health behaviour changes. Miller and Rollnick (2002) argue therefore that resolving ambivalence can in turn be a 'key to change'. Instead of approaching the patient as an individual who does not want to change, by using MI the practitioner focuses on trying to elicit what patients do want, and how they think they might be able to achieve it.

When talking about ambivalence, patients may produce two different kinds of talk reflecting that ambivalence:

- sustain talk – the costs of changing behaviour, or the benefits of not changing;
- change talk – the benefits of changing behaviour, or the costs of not changing.

In MI, the practitioner uses a number of skills to encourage the production of patient change talk. This helps patients to increase their motivation to change their behaviour (Amrhein *et al.* 2003). This does not mean, however, that sustain talk is avoided in MI. Patient autonomy is respected throughout, and sustain talk is accepted as part of the process of exploring ambivalence to change. However, unlike change talk, sustain talk is not purposely elicited by the health professional.

So, how does MI fit into a guiding style of communication? The practitioner can use a number of skills, such as asking open-ended questions, making summaries, and the skilful use of reflective listening both to express empathy and to direct the patient in producing change talk. These skills are used to work collaboratively with the patient, who is the ultimate expert in how and why to make changes to his or her own health behaviour.

One commonly held misconception of MI is that it is a set of techniques that can be inflicted on a patient without genuine empathy and understanding. This is not the case. MI is a clinical *skill* rather than a *tool*. To further define the nature of MI in health care settings, Rollnick *et al.* (2007) describe the *spirit* of MI in health care (or a 'way of being' with a patient), and present four *principles* (or 'conventions guiding practice'). These are discussed in more detail below.

MI SPIRIT

MI spirit is broken down into three components. In practising MI, a practitioner should aim to be:

- collaborative
- evocative
- honouring patient autonomy.

To work collaboratively, the clinician and patient should aim to work together in partnership – for example, the process should perhaps feel like shared decision making rather than the practitioner advocating for change and the patient advocating for no change. A consultation should generally feel like a dance between the patient and the practitioner, rather than a wrestling match. We can see in our example of Mr Green that the practitioner is making all the moves, and Mr Green does not seem to be contributing to the dance very much at all. In fact, his reaction suggests that the practitioner may well have stepped on his toes during the process!

In being evocative, the practitioner elicits the patient's goals, thoughts and feelings about behaviour change, rather than providing information as to how and what the patient should feel about change. Mr Green's clinician appears to have simply given advice as to what to do, rather than trying to understand why Mr Green does not seem to have made any changes.

Honouring patient autonomy involves signifying respect for the patient's autonomy as an individual to make his or her own decisions. For example, Mr Green may have his own ideas about changes he might make if he is allowed to go about them in the way he wants to, in his own time. It is also entirely possible that Mr Green does not want to make any changes. Despite the fact that this is not the best option for his well-being, the practitioner has to accept that Mr Green has made that decision. The ultimate decision about change lies with Mr Green, and Mr Green only.

Later in this chapter, I will be talking about a number of skills and strategies you can use in MI. However, it is most important to get the spirit right – without the spirit, the strategies simply won't work. One study in particular has shown that the single most important factor in influencing behaviour change is the clinician's use of interpersonal skills (Najavitis and Crits-Christoph 2000). In studies where practitioner characteristics have been systematically evaluated and effects found, more favourable outcomes have been associated with the degree of empathy shown by the practitioner towards the client (Miller *et al.* 1993).

MI PRINCIPLES

Rollnick *et al.* (2007) have recently adapted the description of MI principles from the original method to health care contexts. They are described by the acronym RULE:

- Resist the righting reflex.
- Understand your patient's motivations.
- Listen to your patient.
- Empower your patient.

Resisting the righting reflex

The 'righting reflex' refers to our natural urge as human beings to put things right. For example, if we see that somebody is about to accidentally step out into the path of an oncoming car it is natural to hold them back. Bearing in mind our example of Mr Green, it is clear that the clinician is trying to prevent him from coming to any further harm associated with his diabetes and health behaviours. By providing information and advice in the face of Mr Green's apparent resistance to change, the practitioner is hoping to save him from himself, creating a feeling of wrestling rather than dancing. By avoiding this righting reflex, practitioners can instead 'roll with resistance' (Miller and Rollnick 2002), and continue with the dance minus the wrestling. Rolling with resistance is best described as 'going along with what the patient says for a bit' while demonstrating understanding for resistance as a means of reducing it (for example, by saying something like 'You think I'm going to try to force you to do things you're not happy with').

Understand your patient's motivations

This involves listening carefully to your patient's reasons for and against change. What is it that makes them ambivalent about change? Listen carefully to their sustain talk and their change talk, as this will give you more information about why patients are where they are at, at the current time. For example, why does Mr Green's busy life make it more difficult to effect health behaviour changes? What kinds of things hold him back? If he was going to make some changes, how might he go about it? The health professional whom Mr Green saw might have better spent his or her time asking these kinds of questions, rather than telling him what he should do and how he should do it.

Listen to your patient

Often it seems as if listening is a passive process. However, in MI we aim to demonstrate to patients that we have listened carefully to what they have said by using active listening (described below). Doing this is not simply reflecting back the content of what a patient has said in parrot fashion – it is trying to deduce the *meaning* behind what has been said. For example, when Mr Green says 'I'm a busy man, if I had the time to go out and exercise I would have done it by now', an appropriate response might be something like: 'It sounds as though you are fed up with people telling you to get more exercise.'

Empower your patient

As discussed above, if you feel that you will be successful in making changes, you are more likely to achieve your goals than if you doubt yourself. One important thing to do to that end is to help patients feel that change is something they can do, by recognising and reinforcing strengths that they have, and drawing out from (rather than imposing on) them what they think they can do to improve their health. For example, we might say to Mr Green: 'So, despite being really busy and finding it hard to manage your diet, you still managed to take all your medication correctly since the last time we saw you. What other kinds of things do you think you might be able to do to help with your diabetes management?'

USING MI IN PRACTICE

The spirit and principles of MI illustrate to us that our way of being with people, and our approach to behaviour change, are just as – if not more – important than any communication skills and strategies that we might incorporate into our practice. Skills and strategies will be discussed in the next section, but just to recap, when we are practising MI, we need to remember a few things:

- We cannot make somebody else change. The patient is in control of what he or she does, not the practitioner.
- The patient is the *expert* in knowing which changes he or she is more likely to be able to make, which ones fit in with life, how the patient might go about them, and how to cope if things do not go according to plan.
- Establish a good rapport. Don't try to coerce the patient or make judgements.
- Allow patients to resolve their own ambivalence – do not try to resolve it for them.

- Dance, don't wrestle. If you feel as if you are wrestling, this should be a signal that the rapport with the patient is taking a turn for the worst, and steps should be taken to remedy this (see 'Rolling with resistance' on p. 83).

To explore ambivalence about behaviour change with a patient, we need to be curious. To be able to demonstrate that we understand how the patient feels about change, we need to listen carefully to patients and encourage them to describe their feelings. We also need to avoid the urge to tell patients what they should do without their permission. So far, I have talked a lot about our way of being with a patient. The other half of the story is how we actually 'do MI', and using some of the skills and strategies associated with it.

MI SKILLS

Building on the spirit and principles of MI, the clinician can make use of a number of communication skills in the consultation to help patients explore and resolve their ambivalence about behaviour change. Some of them might already be familiar to you, as they are skills that can be used in many different situations – they are not exclusive to MI. For more detailed descriptions of these skills, take a look at Rollnick *et al.* (2007), and/or Miller and Rollnick (2002) and Rollnick *et al.* (1999).

Open vs. closed questioning

Closed questions are those that encourage brief answers, whereas open questions encourage longer answers. Using Mr Green as an example, a closed question might be 'Do you drink when you go out to your pub quizzes?', whereas an open question would be 'How do you feel about your drinking on quiz nights?' Using mainly open rather than closed questions is important in practising MI, because it encourages patients to explore how they feel about a particular behaviour. Open questions are also helpful from the clinicians' point of view, because it helps them to gain a deeper understanding of how the patient feels about making changes.

There are, of course, times where closed questions are necessary, and can be asked skilfully. However, given that the aim of MI is to help patients explore and resolve ambivalence, closed questions should be kept to a minimum to encourage this kind of exploration.

Active listening

Asking too many questions could lead to the patient feeling a little interrogated, and this might increase resistance in the consultation. How can we avoid this? Another way of demonstrating understanding and encouraging the patient to elaborate is through the use of *reflective listening*, one of the most important skills used in MI.

Reflective listening is done through a series of statements, not questions (i.e. the practitioner's intonation must go *downward* at the end of a statement, not upward as at the end of a question). It takes practice to get used to making these statements, but statements have the advantage of being less interrogative and in turn reduce the risk of confrontation. Generally, when using MI, you should aim to use a ratio of two or three reflective listening statements for each question (Miller and Rollnick 2002), as this may help to prevent resistance/confrontational behaviour within the consultation.

By making listening an active process, the clinician can demonstrate that he or she has understood what the patient has said. This involves making a statement in reply to what the patient has just said, and bridges the gap between the practitioner's understanding and what the patient is saying or meaning (see Figure 5.1).

Two broad kinds of reflection may be used within a consultation:

- *content reflections* – short summaries of what the patient has said;
- *meaning reflections* – reflections of what the patient has meant.

For example, if Mr Green said something like 'I wish I could get my blood sugars under control. I want to be well', a *content reflection* of this statement would be something like 'You see a connection between your diabetes control and your health'. A possible *meaning reflection* could be 'Your health is important to you and you want to do whatever you can to be healthy'. Both statements encourage

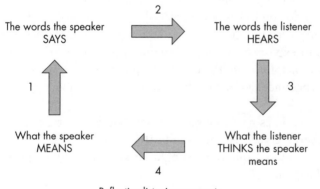

Reflective listening connects
the bottom two processes (4).

Figure 5.1 Active listening

the patient to elaborate further about their reasons, and in turn explore their ambivalence.

As well as reflections, another way to demonstrate understanding and encourage exploration of ambivalence is by using *summaries*. These are lengthier than reflections, and are conducted periodically through the consultation. They can be used to bring together all the things the patient has said regarding a particular issue, to link some things a patient has said with other things he or she has said at another point in the session, or to bring a discussion to a close.

Reflections and summaries are useful tools. As well as demonstrating understanding, they can be used to highlight what patients perceive to be the benefits of changing and the costs of staying the same, and then encouraging them to elaborate on these benefits and costs further. They may also be used to affirm patients, by highlighting their strengths, supporting their achievements and demonstrating appreciation for what they have already managed to do well.

Rolling with resistance

There are times when discussions about behaviour change may lead to resistance – a patient, for example, may disagree with what has been suggested, or become defensive about his or her behaviour. One of the principles of MI is to 'roll with resistance', or rather to respond to resistance with understanding, rather than counter-argument. Rolling with resistance may be done in several ways. The use of reflective listening statements usually helps, as these encourage patients to tell the clinician how they are feeling and why, which in itself can lower resistance.

As we have seen above, resistance often occurs when patients feel that their freedom is being taken away (Brehm 1966). One thing a clinician can do is to reassure patients that they are free to make their own choices, and that they are under no obligation to make changes to their behaviour. For example, the clinician could say to Mr Green: 'I'm not here to force you to change. It's entirely up to you whether you decide to make any changes.'

It can also help to 'shift focus' by acknowledging that the patient is obviously not happy to talk about a particular issue. For example, the practitioner may say to Mr Green: 'It sounds like you aren't really very happy to talk about your diet at the moment. What would you prefer to talk about instead today?'

Resistance may also arise if the clinician has misunderstood how ready the patient is to change. Should this be the case, it can be useful to go back and reassess the patient's readiness (see MI strategies below).

MI STRATEGIES

As well as using communication skills in MI practice, there are a number of strategies that may be used within the consultation. These can be useful in encouraging the exploration of ambivalence, emphasising personal choice and autonomy, and eliciting change talk. For more guidance on the skilful use of these strategies, take a look at Rollnick *et al.* (1999).

Agenda setting and permission seeking

Given that lack of choice in talking about behaviour change can be one of the things that can increase resistance, it is a good idea to encourage patients to be active in choosing to talk about behaviour change. After all, talking about behaviour change should ultimately be the patient's choice.

The first thing the practitioner can do to this end is to ask permission to talk about the behaviour with the patient, rather than just telling the patient that today there will be a discussion about his or her health behaviour. Perhaps saying to Mr Green 'I'm just wondering if it would be all right to have a quick chat with you about your diet in relation to your diabetes. Would that be OK?', rather than simply telling him what to do, might help him feel a little more in control.

In motivational interviewing, the patient is encouraged to suggest what behaviour changes they would like to talk about. This is particularly important if there are a number of different lifestyle issues to be addressed. For example, Mr Green could benefit from making some changes to his diet, taking more exercise, and cutting down on his alcohol intake.

It is often easier to make changes gradually, rather than trying to make a number of substantial changes all in one go. Achieving small changes can increase a person's 'self-efficacy' – their belief in their own ability to make changes (Bandura 1995). Patients are more likely to feel able to make other changes if they have already succeeded with one small change. Starting where patients feel most comfortable, and encouraging them to suggest what area they would like to talk about, is useful both for helping patients to feel more in control of talking about behaviour change, and for starting where they feel most ready to make changes.

So, how can we encourage patients to set the agenda? After all, this might be something they are not used to in a consultation.

This can be approached through the use of open questions, such as: 'There are a number of different things we can talk about today, Mr Green. What is it that you would like to talk to me about today?'

One clinical tool that can help with this task is an 'agenda-setting chart' (Rollnick *et al.* 1999), which contains a number of circles containing picture representations of different lifestyle factors, and some blank circles. The blank circles are for other factors to be inserted by the patient. This means that sometimes the practitioner needs to be prepared for the patient to raise issues that have not previously been expected – for example, perhaps Mr Green is concerned about how the level of stress in his life is currently affecting his diabetes, rather than what he is eating at the moment.

Exploring how the patient feels about change

As we have seen, how ready the patient feels about change can impact directly on his or her motivation to make changes, so spending some time exploring those reasons with the patient is important.

One way this can be achieved within clinical practice is by exploring how important patients feel it is to change their behaviour, and how confident he or she feels in achieving it. Asking 'scaling questions' to do this can be useful. This involves asking patients, on a scale of 0–10, how important it is for them to change a particular behaviour, and then to ask, on the same scale, how confident they feel about successfully making that change. Following on from this, there is the opportunity to ask why they have given themselves this score and not a higher or lower number, or indeed what they think would help them to move up the scale in terms of importance and/or confidence.

Of course, you can do this without asking scaling questions. Importance and confidence could equally be assessed by the use of skilful, open questions, such as: 'How important would you say it is for you to make changes to your diet, Mr Green?' and 'If you made the decision that you were going to change what you eat, how confident are you that you would succeed?'

Another way for patients to explore how they feel about making changes is to help them identify what they like/dislike about their current behaviour, and what they feel they would gain/lose from changing. This is an ideal opportunity for the clinician to elicit change talk from the patient and to reinforce it through reflective listening.

Exchanging information

Obviously, within health care consultations, there are times when patients need information or advice. Perhaps they need to know something concerning their safety or wellbeing, and have asked you for information on what they should do, or they have misunderstood something with regard to their care or recovery.

Information giving within health care is usually a process in which the patient is a passive recipient. Using Mr Green as an example, the healthcare professional might have said something like 'Your HbA1c is still at 10.2. Really, we need to get it down to about 6.5. You need to start taking more care of yourself and eating fewer convenience foods – get a little more fruit and vegetables into your diet. If you don't, then you are putting yourself at risk of complications. You could go blind! I'm sure you don't want that to happen.' This has the advantage of being direct and to the point. However, on the down side, Mr Green might know all this already, or perhaps he does not see how this is relevant to him. It also makes the assumption that Mr Green will just take the advice and do as he is told. We know this is not the case with ambivalent patients, because Mr Green has been back time and again, and has still not implemented any of the advice he has been given.

When taking an MI approach, information is *exchanged* with patients rather than simply given to them, using the 'elicit–provide–elicit' method. This involves, first, finding out what the patient knows already, providing information (after asking if the patient is happy for you to do this), and then finding out what the patient has made of that information. An example of this might be:

Elicit: 'So Mr Green, how much do you know about the complications of diabetes?'
Provide: 'Would it be OK if I told you a little bit more about that?'
Elicit: 'So, what do you think that might mean for you and your diabetes?'

Exchanging information in this way can encourage the patient to actively think about how the information given applies to their self as an individual, and it can even save the clinician time, as it prevents the provision of information that the patient already knows about. The information is given in a neutral manner, and builds on the patient's existing knowledge. Leaving the interpretation of the facts to patients helps them to recognise what the personal relevance of the information is – rather than listening to the reasons why the practitioner thinks this information is relevant.

Talking about making changes

If a patient indicates that he or she is ready to make changes, the most useful course of action is to elicit from the patient what changes he or she feels able to make. Focusing on small changes that feel achievable can help the patient to feel more confident of success, and more able to face other changes (Bandura 1995). If major changes need to be made, it may be easier for the patient to break these changes down into smaller tasks, rather than trying to do them all at once.

The health professional who Mr Green saw no doubt has years of experience in clinical practice and knows exactly what he needs to do to achieve better diabetes control. However, as it is Mr Green who has to make these changes, he is the expert, as he knows what will work best for him. The patient should be an active decision maker, rather than a passive recipient of information and advice.

How might we go about drawing this out of Mr Green? Using some good open questions such as 'What sorts of things do you think you might be able to do?' might be helpful to start things off. This does not mean that the health professional cannot offer possible courses of action to the patient – Mr Green might even ask for advice about what he could do. Before making a suggestion, however, it is a good idea to ask permission, and to emphasise that it is up to the patient to decide if he or she thinks it will be useful. For example, the clinician might say something like: 'Trying to fit exercise into your everyday life, so that you don't have to change your routine too much, sounds like it might be the most workable for you. Some of the patients I see say that they try to take a 10-minute walk after their dinner in the evening. Do you think that's something that might work for you?'

Another thing that can be helpful is to encourage patients to think about previous attempts to change their behaviour. For example, asking Mr Green what has worked well before, what kinds of things did not work, and why, might help him to think about different things that he might try to change this time.

WHAT IS THE EVIDENCE FOR MI?

A number of recent systematic reviews have presented growing evidence for the effectiveness of MI as an intervention.

The strongest evidence is in the treatment of drug and alcohol misuse (Dunn *et al.* 2001; Burke *et al.* 2003; Hettema *et al.* 2005). As MI is still a relatively new method, and it entered the general health care arena much later than the addictions field, the evidence for MI within health care settings is more limited, although it has shown much promise. Rubak *et al.* (2005) conducted a systematic review of 72 randomised controlled trials in health care settings, and found that MI interventions had a significant effect on reducing BMI, cholesterol, systolic blood pressure, blood alcohol content and standard ethanol content, although not on the number of cigarettes per day in smokers or HbA1c in people with diabetes. Vasilaki *et al.* (2006) systematically reviewed studies that used brief alcohol interventions based on MI, and concluded that MI was effective in reducing alcohol consumption in the short term with mainly risky (rather than alcohol-dependent) drinkers. A recent systematic review by Knight *et al.* (2006) into the effects of MI interventions on physical activity concluded that these interventions do appear to increase exercise uptake among patients, although the poor quality of trials made this hard to determine, with just eight studies being included in the review as a result – mirroring the findings of previous reviews that have attempted to look at MI in relation to specific health behaviours (Dunn *et al.* 2001; Burke *et al.* 2003; Hettema *et al.* 2005). To enhance the quality of such trials of MI, more attention is being focused on the quality of the intervention actually delivered by practitioners in a number of different contexts, resulting in the development of instruments to measure practitioner skill in delivering MI (Lane *et al.* 2005; Madson *et al.* 2005, Moyers *et al.* 2005).

DEVELOPING MI SKILLS

In this chapter, we have explored the process of behaviour change and looked at the issue of patients who are ambivalent to change, and what might be helpful. We have looked at the spirit and principles of MI, the skills and strategies we might want to employ while using an MI approach, and the evidence for using MI in practice.

However, this chapter has only touched on the basics of MI. You may feel that you would like some more detailed description of how you can incorporate this into your practice, and indeed to have some formal training to develop your own MI skills.

Publications such as Rollnick *et al.* (1999, 2007) and Miller and Rollnick (2002) describe the processes outlined above in much more detail, and you may find them useful.

There are many training courses available on MI. The Motivational Interviewing Network of Trainers (MINT) advertises courses being run by its members all over the world, and lists MI trainers who are willing to deliver MI training on its website: www.motivationalinterview.org. You will also find many other helpful resources on this website about learning MI, including instruments to assess clinical skills in MI.

KEY POINTS

- There are many factors that may affect an individual's motivation to change.
- Many patients are ambivalent about making changes.
- MI is a refined form of a guiding style of communication that aims to help patients explore and resolve ambivalence to change.
- MI has been used in a range of different contexts involving behaviour change.
- There are many skills and strategies a practitioner can use in MI, but it is most important to adhere to the spirit and principles.
- A recent systematic review has demonstrated that MI in health care contexts has been associated with positive patient outcomes.
- There are resources you can access to try to help you learn more about MI, and develop your own skills.
- No matter how much you try, you cannot *make* somebody change!

FURTHER AREAS TO CONSIDER

- How useful do you think MI could be to you in clinical practice?
- How can you best adhere to the spirit and principles of MI?
- How can you best develop your skills in MI?
- To what extent do you think you could integrate MI into your own clinical practice?
- What are the challenges to implementing MI in clinical practice? What kinds of things could help you?

CHAPTER 6

HOW TO IDENTIFY A PERSON WITH A LONG-TERM CONDITION

OVERVIEW

A definition of what a long-term condition (LTC) constitutes and what conditions are regarded as long term has been supplied in Chapter 1. This chapter is a practical guide to straightforward diagnostic criteria (where these exist) of some of the conditions that constitute an LTC (e.g. diabetes, asthma, chronic obstructive pulmonary disease (COPD)). For conditions that have more complex diagnostic criteria such as cardiovascular disease, epilepsy or arthritis, a brief overview is provided with reference to appropriate texts. The aim is not to supply detailed manuals on every LTC but to discuss general principles relating to diagnosis.

INTRODUCTION

Previous chapters have discussed the varying types of conditions that may be considered to be long term. These range greatly in type, presentation and prevalence. In Chapter 2 the WHO (2002b) definition of a chronic condition was provided to demonstrate that the term 'LTC' should no longer be confined to conditions of greatest prevalence or ones that lead to the highest mortality rates, but should include any condition, physical/structural or mental, that impacts on health, will worsen without health care intervention and/or behaviour change on the part of the patient and for which there is no defined cure at the present time.

This chapter will provide diagnostic criteria, where available, relating to some of the LTCs discussed in Chapter 2 to offer the reader some practical guidance regarding appropriate screening, detection and diagnosis of an LTC. The criteria used are those currently recommended in the UK. Some reference will be made to the differences in other countries, particularly regarding diagnostic criteria, but users who are not UK based should ensure that they consult the correct criteria for their own country and not rely solely on those provided in this book. You should also be aware that diagnostic criteria are subject to regular updating; what is accurate today may be out of date next year. To this end the sources of the criteria will be provided and the reader should ensure access to these sources before making a firm diagnosis of an LTC. Where firm diagnostic criteria do not currently exist the signs and symptoms of the condition will be discussed, although again the reader should be aware that diagnosis is a complex art and appropriate medical professionals should always be involved in discussions relating to individual diagnosis. Although general treatment principles for LTCs have been discussed throughout this book and examples of care using case studies will be provided in Chapter 9, specific treatment for individual conditions is not discussed and readers should refer to appropriate evidence-based guidelines (details in Chapter 8) for more precise treatment procedures.

DIABETES MELLITUS

There are currently five clinical categories of disordered glucose homeostasis:

- type 1 diabetes
- type 2 diabetes
- impaired glucose tolerance/impaired fasting glucose
- gestational diabetes
- other specific types: including rare forms such as the genetic condition maturity-onset diabetes in the young (MODY), other genetic and endocrine conditions affecting the pancreas, disorders of the exocrine pancreas, drug and chemical-related causes.

(BMA 2004)

The following signs and symptoms should alert health care professionals to the possibility of diabetes:

- weight loss
- polydipsia (excessive thirst)

- polyuria (increased urine production)
- incontinence
- tiredness/lethargy
- recurrent infections (e.g. thrush, cystitis, balanitis)
- mood changes
- altered vision
- foot ulceration
- delayed wound healing
- ketoacidosis.

Differentiation between types

Type 1 diabetes is classically a disease of the young but can occur at any age; onset is generally rapid and presentation acute. Causation in the majority of cases is an auto-immune process which destroys the insulin-producing pancreatic beta cells. Both genetic and environmental factors have been implicated as important factors in the initiation of the auto-immune process, with viruses often acting as a trigger (BMA 2004). The process of pancreatic beta cell destruction normally takes place over a few weeks with symptoms becoming apparent as glucose levels build up due to the lack of insulin. Type 1 diabetes should be suspected in a patient of any age who presents with sudden weight loss and raised blood glucose. The presence of ketonuria in the absence of fasting can aid in the differentiation between type 1 and type 2 diabetes (BMA 2004).

In adults with suspected type 1 diabetes where classical symptoms are present, diagnosis can be confirmed by a single laboratory glucose measurement; this should be repeated if classical symptoms are not present (NICE 2004b). A full medical, environmental, cultural and educational assessment should be performed to develop an individualised and culturally appropriate care plan, including choice of insulin and insulin regime, self monitoring of blood glucose and education relating to dietary management and lifestyle (NICE 2004b). This should be negotiated between the professional team and the person with type 1 diabetes and implemented without inappropriate delay (NICE 2004b). Without treatment diabetic ketoacidosis (DKA) (see Chapter 2) may develop which can lead to coma and eventually death. Additional symptoms that indicate DKA include:

- vomiting
- stomach pain
- rapid breathing
- increased pulse rate
- sleepiness.

Type 2 diabetes is generally preceded by an asymptomatic period of impaired glucose tolerance, which is characterised by a response to an oral glucose challenge that is not normal, but is not diagnostic of diabetes (BMA 2004). Type 2 diabetes is the most common type of diabetes, accounting for 90 per cent of all cases of diabetes, and is frequently undiagnosed, with perhaps as many as half the number of individuals who have this type of diabetes being unaware of their condition (BMA 2004). Although type 2 diabetes has characteristically been thought of as a condition affecting the middle-aged and elderly, it is increasingly being detected in younger people, including children. The possibility of type 2 diabetes should be suspected in younger people presenting with symptoms of diabetes who are obese, have a family history of type 2 diabetes or are of non-white ethnicity (NICE 2004b). The risk factors relating to development of type 2 diabetes include obesity, particularly central abdominal obesity, reduced physical activity and genetic predisposition (including ethnicity), as well as intrauterine factors. Insulin resistance, initial hyperinsulinaemia and later beta cell destruction resulting in reduced insulin levels are well recognised in the pathogenesis of type 2 diabetes (BMA 2004). The distinction between type 1 and type 2 diabetes can, however, be blurred with some patients presenting with type 2 having an incomplete form of type 1 disease. Type 1 diabetes should be considered if ketonuria is detected or if weight loss is marked (NICE 2004b).

The WHO recommendations for definition and diagnosis of diabetes mellitus and intermediate hyperglycaemia were reviewed in 2006. The issues discussed at the time included whether the current diabetes diagnostic criteria should be changed, how normal plasma glucose levels, impaired glucose tolerance and impaired fasting glucose should be defined and what tests used to define glycaemic status. Based on data available at the time and current recommendations, a number of recommendations were made and these are summarised below:

- Current WHO diagnostic criteria of fasting plasma glucose (FPG) $\geq$ 7.0mmol/l (126mg/dl) *or* 2–h plasma glucose $\geq$ 11.1mmol/l (200mg/dl) should be maintained as these criteria identify a group with significantly increased premature mortality and increased risk of microvascular and cardiovascular complications.
- 'Normoglycaemia' should be used for glucose levels associated with low risk of developing diabetes or cardiovascular disease.
- The current WHO recommendation for impaired glucose tolerance (IGT) should remain at present, although consideration should be given to replacing this by an overall risk assessment for diabetes and cardiovascular disease, including a measure of glucose as a continuous variable.
- The fasting plasma glucose cut-point for impaired fasting glucose (IFG) should remain at 6.1mmol/l, and consideration should be given to replacing this by an overall risk assessment for diabetes and cardiovascular disease, including a measure of glucose as a continuous variable.
- Venous plasma glucose should be the standard method for measuring and reporting glucose concentrations in blood, although, since many under-

resourced countries use capillary sampling, conversion values for post-load glucose values are provided within the document, and fasting values are identical.

- The oral glucose tolerance test (OGTT) should be retained as a diagnostic test, and since FPG fails to identify 30 per cent of undiagnosed cases, OGTT is the only means of identifying people with IGT. OGTT is often required to exclude or confirm abnormal glucose tolerance in asymptomatic people. An OGTT should be used in individuals with fasting plasma glucose 6.1–6.9mmol/l (110–125mg/dl) to determine glucose tolerance status.
- Currently HbA1c is not considered a suitable diagnostic test for diabetes or intermediate hyperglycaemia.

(WHO 2006b)

Table 6.1 summarises the WHO (2006b) recommendations.

Diagnosis of diabetes requires careful substantiation with retesting on another day unless the person is symptomatic and the plasma glucose is unequivocally elevated.

Although both the American Diabetic Asoociation (ADA) and the previous 1999 WHO criteria for diagnosing diabetes defined normal plasma glucose levels the current WHO criteria recommends that since there are insufficient data to accurately define normal glucose levels, the term 'normoglycaemia' should be used for glucose levels associated with low risk of developing diabetes or cardiovascular disease; that is, levels below those used to define intermediate hyperglycaemia.

Table 6.1 WHO recommendations for definition and diagnosis of diabetes mellitus and intermediate hyperglycaemia

---

Diabetes mellitus
Fasting plasma glucose ≥7.0mmol/l (126mg/dl)
or
2–h plasma glucose* ≥11.1mmol/l (200mg/dl)

Impaired glucose tolerance (IGT)
Fasting plasma glucose <7.0mmol/l (126mg/dl)
and
2–h plasma glucose* ≥7.8 and <11.1mmol/l (140mg/dl and 200mg/dl)

Impaired fasting glucose (IFG)
Fasting plasma glucose 6.1 to 6.9mmol/l (110mg/dl to 125mg/dl)
and (if measured)
2–h plasma glucose* <7.8mmol/l (140mg/dl)

- Venous plasma glucose two hours after ingestion of 75g oral glucose load
- If two-hour plasma glucose is not measured, status is uncertain, as diabetes or IGT cannot be excluded.

(WHO 2006b, p. 3)

Following confirmation of diagnosis a full clinical assessment should be performed prior to an agreed treatment plan being initiated. This should include full medical examination, body mass index and waist measurement, blood pressure, cardiovascular risk assessment, referral for retinal photography, foot examination including peripheral vascular assessment, urinalysis, and blood tests including: HbA1c (glycated haemoglobin) as a marker, urea and electrolytes, estimated glomerular filtration rate (eGFR), liver function, thyroid function, and lipid profile.

CARDIOVASCULAR DISEASE

Cardiovascular disease (CVD), as noted in Chapter 2, is an umbrella term for all diseases of the heart and circulation including: angina, myocardial infarction, heart failure, arrhythmia (including atrial fibrillation), hypertension, thrombosis, cerebral vascular disease and peripheral vascular disease. It would be impossible to provide in full detail diagnostic criteria for all these conditions in the confines of this chapter. Indeed, many of the above present initially as acute conditions that warrant emergency treatment and initial management in secondary, rather than primary care. Instead, some of the signs and symptoms relating to those conditions suitable for diagnosis in the primary care setting will be discussed.

Angina

Clinical Knowledge Summaries (CKS) (2007b) provide the following information relating to the diagnosis of angina:

- Angina pain is characterised by pain in the chest, brought on by effort or emotion and relieved by rest.
- It is often described as a great weight on the chest, squeezing, crushing or a vice-like grip. Others may describe it as discomfort.
- Although typical presentation is symmetrical central chest pain, some people complain of pain in the neck or jaw or of pain radiating down the arm.
- Breathlessness on exertion is typical of angina; for some people this is the only symptom.

(adapted from CKS 2007b)

People with suspected angina should in the majority of cases be referred for specialist confirmation and assessment. History should include characteristics of the pain, additional symptoms (e.g. breathlessness), precursors of symptoms, type of physical activity that causes pain, stability of symptoms, past medical history and family history. Physical examination should include: height, weight, BMI (body mass index), waist circumference measurement, blood pressure, pulse rate, chest auscultation for murmurs, and examination for signs of hyper-lipidaemia, vascular disease, anaemia and hyperthyroidism. Investigations should include: blood tests; full blood count, serum creatinine or eGFR, lipid profile, fasting blood glucose and thyroid function, 12 lead electrocardiograph (ECG), and exercise stress testing unless this has already been carried out or is contraindicated or inappropriate. Diagnosis should exclude other cardiac and non-cardiac causes of chest pain (CKS 2007b).

Hypertension

Hypertension is a well-known risk factor for cardiovascular disease; assessment of people with hypertension should concentrate on total risk of cardiovascular disease and not just blood pressure alone (British Hypertension Society (BHS) Guidelines: Williams *et al.* 2004). In 95 per cent of people hypertension has no known cause (primary hypertension), while 5 per cent have hypertension secondary to an underlying condition. For those with secondary hypertension, treatment of the underlying condition can result in improved blood pressure. Hypertension (in people without diabetes) is defined as a sustained systolic blood pressure of > = 140 mmHg or as a sustained diastolic blood pressure of > = 90 mmHg. A sustained blood pressure is defined as an initial raised blood pressure measurement persisting at two or more subsequent consultations; an average of two readings at each consultation should guide the decision to treat. Measurements should be taken in both arms at first consultation, the arm with the highest reading used for future measurement. Ideally when a blood pressure of > = 140/90 mmHg is recorded at first consultation several readings should be taken over several weeks. Monthly intervals are generally suitable; people with severe hypertension and increased cardiovascular risk should be evaluated more urgently.

People with hypertension should have a thorough history taken and a physical examination; tests should be limited to urinalysis for blood and protein, serum creatinine, electrolytes and eGFR, fasting blood glucose and lipid profile (Williams *et al.* 2004). All people with high blood pressure, borderline or high normal blood pressure should be advised on lifestyle modifications. Thresholds and guidance for anti-hypertensive drug treatment are set out in the NICE (2006a) guidelines. Treatment thresholds are lower for those with diabetes, complication of hypertension or target organ damage or in people whose ten-year CVD risk, estimated by the Joint British Societies risk charts, is > = 20%.

Heart failure

CKS (2006a) notes that accurate clinical diagnosis of heart failure is difficult, due to clinical signs and symptoms being poorly predictive; they further add that a history of myocardial infarction and presence of multiple signs/symptoms increases the likelihood of a diagnosis of heart failure being correct. NICE (2003, p. 4) notes that evaluation of heart failure involves excluding other conditions and

> requires consideration of the underlying abnormality of the heart, the severity of the syndrome, the aetiology, precipitating and exacerbating factors, identification of concomitant disease relevant to the management, and an estimation of prognosis.

Symptoms include breathlessness, fatigue, ankle swelling, orthopnoea and paroxysmal nocturnal dyspnoea. The signs noted as most predictive of heart failure are: laterally displaced apex beat, elevated jugular venous pressure (JVP) and third heart sound (gallop rhythm). Other possible but less predictive signs may include tachycardia, lung crepitations, oedema and hepatomegaly (CKS 2006a). Tests should include:

*   twelve lead ECG and /or natriuretic peptides (where available), with imaging by echocardiography if one of these is abnormal;
*   chest x-ray;
*   urinalysis;
*   peak flow or spirometry;
*   blood tests to include: U&Es, creatinine, FBC, TFTs, LFTs, fasting glucose and lipid profile.

(NICE 2003; CKS 2006a)

Other causes of shortness of breath, peripheral oedema and any other conditions causing similar symptoms should be eliminated before a definitive diagnosis is made.

Peripheral vascular/arterial disease

Peripheral vascular disease (PVD) or peripheral arterial disease (PAD) is caused by atheroma (fatty deposits) in the walls of the arteries leading to insufficient blood flow to the muscles and other tissues (Scottish Intercollegiate Guidelines Network (SIGN) 2006). Although the condition can present as asymptomatic, intermittent claudication – leg pain and weakness brought on by walking and relieved by rest – is the most common symptom. Patients with PAD are at increased cardiovascular risk and have an increased mortality risk. The Fontaine classification (SIGN 2006) describes PAD as follows:

- Stage I: asymptomatic
- Stage II: intermittent claudication
- Stage III: rest pain/nocturnal pain
- Stage IV: necrosis/gangrene.

SIGN (2006) provides the following guidance to diagnosis of PAD at Stage II. Diagnosis should be based on clinical history, examination of peripheral pulses (femoral/popliteal/foot) and abdominal palpation for aneurysm. Ankle brachial pressure index (ABPI) should be measured at rest by properly trained practitioners, using a sphygmomanometer and handheld Doppler device. A resting ABPI < 0.9 is considered abnormal, although normal ABPI at rest, in combination with classic symptoms, should necessitate further investigation. Critical limb ischaemia is associated with ABPI < 0.5. In people with heavily calcified vessels, such as those with diabetes and advanced chronic renal failure, care should be taken when interpreting readings, as vessels are likely to be incompressible and results artificially high. Young and otherwise healthy adults presenting prematurely with claudication should be referred to exclude entrapment syndromes and other rare disorders.

CHRONIC KIDNEY DISEASE

The SIGN (2008) clinical guideline *Diagnosis and Management of Chronic Kidney Disease* provides clear directions on identification of individuals more likely to develop chronic kidney disease (CKD), diagnostic criteria, how to reduce the risk of developing CKD and recommendations on how to slow progression of CKD and reduce risk of cardiovascular disease for adults over 18 years. Management of patients with end stage renal failure, acute kidney disease and features suggestive of a primary renal diagnosis are excluded from the guideline. SIGN (2008) states that all patients with evidence of persisting kidney damage for more than 90 days are defined as having CKD. They also note that epidemiology has revealed an association between a number of clinical characteristics (diabetes mellitus, hypertension, CVD, smoking, age, chronic use of non-steroidal anti-inflammatory drugs (NSAIDS), obesity, socio-economic status) and development of CKD, although for some associations evidence is weak.

The recommendations include regular surveillance of patients with diabetes and annual renal function assessment in people taking anti-hypertensives and lipid-lowering therapy, or with other known risk factors (SIGN 2008). Where initial abnormality (through urine dipstick/measure of renal function or kidney structural abnormality) is detected, during surveillance, or through

Table 6.2 Stages of chronic kidney disease

Stage	GFR	Description
1	90+	Normal kidney function but urine findings or structural abnormalities or genetic trait pointing to kidney disease
2	60–89	Mildly reduced kidney function and other findings (as for stage 1) pointing to kidney disease
3	30–59	Moderately reduced kidney function
4	15–29	Severely reduced kidney function
5	<15	Very severe, or end stage kidney failure (sometimes call established renal failure)

(adapted from Renal Association 2007)

incidental testing, a full clinical evaluation should be performed. This should include history taking, examination and confirmation of initial observations, with urine sent for protein quantifications. Where relevant symptoms are present a renal tract ultrasound should be arranged. If acute or 'acute on chronic' disease is suspected, urgent repeat blood tests should be arranged and specialist referral made if there is a rapidly progressive decline in kidney function (SIGN 2008).

Chronic kidney disease is defined according to the presence or absence of kidney damage and level of kidney function – irrespective of the type of kidney disease. Stages of kidney disease are based on the American National Kidney Foundation-Kidney Disease Quality Outcomes Initiative (NKF K/DOQI) guidelines (Renal Association 2007). Stage of disease should be based on level of kidney function, irrespective of diagnosis. SIGN (2008) suggests that this classification system should only be used after clinical evaluation and diagnosis of CKD. The stages, based on estimated or measured GFR, are shown in Table 6.2.

The Renal Association (2007) notes that kidney function is normal in stage 1 and minimally reduced in stage 2; the Association also emphasises that stage 2 may be overdiagnosed by eGFR alone. This is due to the potential of the equations used to predict eGFR to give falsely low results in people with near-normal function. They note that diagnosis of stage 2 CKD on the basis of slightly reduced eGFR alone is not recommended in the UK CKD guidelines.

EPILEPSY

Epilepsy is a difficult condition to diagnose, with misdiagnosis common; it is recommended that all adults having a first seizure and children having a first non-febrile seizure should be seen by a specialist medical practitioner or paediatrician with training and expertise in epilepsy (CKS 2006b). This will ensure precise and early diagnosis and treatment initiation appropriate to need. Within primary care it is recommended that where seizure is suspected a full history should be obtained about the event, accompanied by a physical examination, and referral to an epilepsy specialist should be made within two weeks (NICE 2004c). Key symptoms that should be enquired for include: loss of awareness, generalised convulsive movements, drop attacks, transient focal motor attacks or transient focal sensory attacks, facial muscle and eye movements, psychic experiences, and episodic phenomena in sleep (CKS 2006b). Other seizure-related symptoms to enquire for include:

- sudden falls;
- involuntary jerky movements of limbs while awake;
- blank spells;
- unexplained incontinence of urine with loss of awareness, or in sleep;
- odd events occurring in sleep (e.g. fall from bed, jerky movements, automatisms);
- episodes of confused behaviour.

(CKS 2006b)

Specialist diagnosis will include detailed history of the attack and symptoms from the person who experienced the attack and eye witness(es). Electroencephalography (EEG) may be used to support diagnosis, and neuro-imaging may be used to identify structural abnormalities that cause certain epilepsies. Magnetic resonance imaging (MRI) is the imaging investigation of choice.

RESPIRATORY CONDITIONS

Asthma

This section is based on diagnostic criteria in children and adults as detailed in the British Thoracic Society (BTS)/SIGN (2008) guidelines. Although this book mainly concentrates on LTCs in adults, asthma in both adults and children is a common problem seen in the primary care environment and so diagnostic criteria for both are detailed here.

Diagnosis in children

Asthma causes recurrent respiratory systems of wheezing, coughing, difficulty in breathing and chest tightness in children. Wheezing should be distinguished from stridor or rattly breathing and it is important to be aware that there are many causes of wheezing in childhood. Diagnosis of asthma is based on recognising an episodic pattern of signs and symptoms with no alternative explanation.

BTS/SIGN (2008, p. iv3) outlines the clinical features that increase the probability of asthma in children as:

- More than one of the following: wheezing, coughing, difficulty breathing and chest tightness, particularly if these symptoms are frequent or recurrent, worse at night/early in the morning, occur in response to, or are worse after, triggers such as exercise, pets, cold air, emotions or laughter, or occur after colds.
- Personal history of atopic disorder.
- Family history of asthma/atopic disorder.
- Widespread wheeze detected on chest auscultation.
- History of improvement in symptoms or lung function in response to adequate therapy.

A number of factors outlined in the guidelines make a diagnosis of asthma more likely, with family atopy, particularly maternal atopy, the most clearly defined risk factor. Assessment of suspected asthma in children should be based on the presence of key features in the history and examination and careful consideration of alternative diagnoses. BTS/SIGN (2008, p. iv5) advises that based on initial clinical assessment it should be possible to determine the probability of a diagnosis of asthma, and suggests:

- Children with a high probability of asthma should be put straight on to a trial of treatment with response reviewed and further testing arranged for those with poor response.
- Children with a low probability of asthma should be further investigated and referred for specialist assessment.

In children with an intermediate probability of asthma, approaches include: watchful waiting with review, trial of treatment with review, or spirometry and reversibility testing, although this is difficult in cases of children under 5. Normal results on testing, especially if performed when the child is asymptomatic, do not exclude a diagnosis of asthma.

Diagnosis in adults

BTS/SIGN (2008) emphasises that a diagnosis of asthma is made by careful clinical history to determine a characteristic pattern of signs and symptoms and a measure of airflow obstruction, preferably via spirometry, where available. Normal spirometry or peak expiratory flow (PEF) measurements made when a person is not symptomatic do not exclude asthma diagnosis. History should also explore possible causes, including occupational. Clinical features that increase the probability of asthma in adults include:

- More than one of the following: wheezing, breathlessness, chest tightness and coughing, particularly if symptoms are worse at night/early in the morning, or in response to exercise, allergen exposure or cold air, or after taking aspirin or beta blockers.
- History of atopic disorder.
- Family history of asthma/atopic disorder.
- Widespread wheezing detected on chest auscultation.
- Unexplained low FEV1 (forced expiratory volume) or PEF.
- Unexplained peripheral blood eosinophilia.

(BTS/SIGN 2008, p. iv12)

BTS/SIGN (2008, p. iv14) suggest that following diagnosis, based on assessment of symptoms and measure of airflow obstruction, the following treatment should be instigated:

- Patients with a high probability of asthma should be put straight on to a trial of treatment.
- Patients with a low probability of asthma in whom symptoms are thought to point to an alternative diagnosis should be investigated and managed accordingly. Asthma should be reconsidered if there is no response to treatment.

In patients with an intermediate probability of asthma, further investigations should be carried out, including a trial of treatment before diagnosis is confirmed and maintenance treatment established.

Chronic obstructive pulmonary disease

COPD is characterised by airflow obstruction that is usually progressive, not fully reversible and does not change markedly over several months; diagnosis is based on assessment of signs and symptoms with a measure of severity of airflow obstruction (NICE 2004d). NICE (2004d) published the Thorax guideline: *Management of Chronic Obstructive Pulmonary Disease in Adults in Primary and Secondary Care*, which contains the following recommendations relating to diagnosis.

Diagnosis of COPD relies on clinical judgement based on history, physical examination and confirmation of airflow obstruction using spirometry. A diagnosis of COPD should be considered in patients over the age of 35 who have a risk factor (generally smoking) and who present with one or more of the following symptoms:

- exertional breathlessness (graded by the Medical Research Council (MRC)) dyspnoea scale

- chronic cough
- regular sputum production
- frequent winter bronchitis
- wheezing.

Patients in whom a diagnosis of COPD is considered should also be asked about the presence of the following factors:

- weight loss
- effort intolerance
- waking at night
- ankle swelling
- fatigue
- occupational hazards
- chest pain
- haemoptysis.

Chest pain and haemoptysis are uncommon in COPD and raise the possibility of alternative diagnoses (NICE 2004d). Spirometry should be performed at the time of diagnosis and to reconfirm diagnosis where an exceptionally good response to treatment is shown. In addition to spirometry, at initial diagnostic evaluation all patients should have a chest x-ray to exclude other pathologies, a full blood count to identify anaemia or polycythaemia and calculation of BMI. Differentiation between COPD and asthma should be made, based on the history and examination of untreated patients, and on longitudinal observation; routine spirometric reversibility testing as part of the diagnostic process can be unhelpful or misleading (NICE 2004d). Additional investigations may be necessary in some circumstances – see full guidelines (NICE 2004d).

MUSCULOSKELETAL CONDITIONS

Arthritis

Osteoarthritis

Diagnosis of osteoarthritis (OA) is usually made following clinical examination and history taking. The National Collaborating Centre for Chronic Conditions (NCC-CC) (2008) has identified a number of risk factors for OA, including genetic, environmental and occupational factors:

- Genetic factors play a part, particularly for hand, knee and hip (approximately 40 to 60 per cent show genetic factors) although as yet the specific genes responsible remain elusive.

- Age, female sex, obesity, high bone density.
- Biomechanical factors (previous joint injury, occupational, sport injuries), reducing muscle strength or joint misalignment.

The NCC-CC (2008) guideline group provides a clinician's working diagnosis of peripheral joint osteoarthritis as:

- persistent joint pain that is worse with use;
- aged 45 years and over;
- morning stiffness lasting no longer than half an hour.

It further suggests that people meeting this working diagnosis do not generally require radiological or laboratory investigations. Other symptoms that can add to diagnostic certainty if required include: inactivity pain and stiffness known as 'gelling', examination findings of crepitus or bony swelling, radiological evidence and absence of clinical/laboratory evidence of inflammation such as acutely inflamed joints or markers of inflammation. The working diagnosis excludes other joint disorders (such as inflammatory arthritis) and connective tissue disorders; however, the NCC-CC (2008) guideline group reinforces that people with inflammatory arthritis may also have secondary osteoarthritis, in which case parts of the guidelines may also apply to them.

Rheumatoid arthritis

Diagnosis of rheumatoid arthritis (RA) is based on clinical features and investigations. CKS (2005) notes that typical symptoms include pain, stiffness, and swelling of the joints with symptoms often worse in the morning and after inactivity. Symptoms are often accompanied by systemic 'flu-like' symptoms. Rheumatoid arthritis can present as gradual onset mainly affecting the hands and/or feet or as acute onset affecting large joints such as the shoulders and knees with extra articular or systemic features. Symmetrical swelling and tenderness of the small joints of the hands and feet are usually found on examination. CKS (2005) also provides the American College of Rheumatology (ACR) criteria, which it notes are more useful in research than in clinical practice; four out of the seven criteria are considered diagnostic. These are briefly summarised below, and full details may be obtained from CKS (2005) or from the ACR:

- morning stiffness
- arthritis of three or more joint areas observed by a physician
- arthritis of hand joints
- symmetric arthritis
- rheumatoid nodules

- serum rheumatoid factor
- radiographic changes.

(adapted from CKS 2005)

Investigations should support the clinical diagnosis; negative results do not exclude or confirm RA. These include: C-reactive protein (CRP) or erythrocyte sedimentation rate (ESR), full blood count, liver function tests, urinalysis, rheumatoid factor, antinuclear antibodies and radiology (CKS 2005).

Osteoporosis

CKS (2006c) provides the following information relating to diagnosis of osteoporosis. Osteoporosis is generally diagnosed by bone mineral density (BMD), which when measured alone has high specificity but low sensitivity (in the general population 50 per cent of osteoporotic fractures will occur in women considered not to have osteoporosis) for fracture risk. Dual-energy x-ray absorptiometry (DXA) is the recommended gold standard test for BMD. This should be measured at two sites, preferably the lumbar spine and femoral neck, with the prediction of fracture risk based on BMD measurements taken at the femoral neck. Biochemical markers have no role in the diagnosis of osteoporosis. The following people should be referred for measurement of BMD:

- People with a fragility fracture (except women aged over 75 who should be assumed to have osteoporosis and offered treatment).
- People at high risk of osteoporosis (untreated premature menopause, prolonged secondary amenorrhoea, primary hypogonadism, chronic disorders associated with osteoporosis, family history of maternal hip fracture under 75 years of age, BMI < 19, prolonged immobility).
- People with thoracic kyphosis and height loss due to vertebral deformity.
- People with x-ray evidence of osteopenia or vertebral deformity.
- Post-menopausal women with two vertebral fractures.
- People under the age of 65 taking oral corticosteroids for three months or more.
- People who have had a DXA scan of the wrist or heel carried out as a screening process that indicates osteoporosis.

(CKS 2006c)

This chapter has provided an overview of diagnostic criteria and the signs and symptoms associated with many, but by no means all, of the LTCs that often present in primary care. Although diagnosis for some of these will be made and treatment plans instigated in primary care, other LTCs will require more specialist input to ensure that a correct diagnosis is made. No diagnosis should be made without taking a clear history and conducting an appropriate clinical examination.

KEY POINTS

- Diagnosis of a long-term condition should always include careful history taking and clinical examination.
- Where diagnostic criteria exist these should be interpreted with regard to the overall clinical picture; for many LTCs negative investigations do not necessarily rule out a positive diagnosis.
- Differential diagnosis should always be considered, particularly where signs and symptoms vary, or if improvement is not achieved with an appropriate treatment plan.
- Diagnosis for some LTCs can be complex and referral to specialists for firm diagnosis should be made where recommended in the guidelines.

FURTHER AREAS TO CONSIDER

- Which conditions should be referred for specialist investigation?
- Are you aware of the relevant referral procedures in your area?
- Which evidence-based sources are you aware of where you can access diagnostic criteria?
- How do you ensure that you have the relevant skills for history taking/ clinical examination?

CHAPTER 7

EFFECTIVE MANAGEMENT OF PEOPLE WITH A LONG-TERM CONDITION

OVERVIEW

This chapter provides a practical guide on clinical management including issues such as: writing a protocol, registration, recall and review, follow-up appointments, referral criteria and clinical audit mechanisms. Ways of identifying patients in the practice population to ensure registers are up to date are discussed, including how to ensure an effective call/recall system.

INTRODUCTION

So far national and international policies guiding the care and management of people with long-term conditions (LTCs) have been reviewed, along with the key principles relating to care provision, including case management and the importance of self-care. The physical and psychological aspects of living with an LTC have been discussed along with social influences on health. The key principles of behaviour change and motivational interviewing have been introduced and examples provided of how to put these principles into practice. In Chapter 6 signs, symptoms and criteria relating to diagnosis were introduced to ensure that people with LTCs are identified. The importance of IT systems, the use of shared records and the benefits of assistive technology should also not be forgotten. So what next? you may ask. Once diagnosis is established and the type and level of care provision have been determined, how do you actually implement all this? How can you ensure that the service you provide to people with LTCs runs smoothly and efficiently, that care is not duplicated or essential elements missed and that people are not lost to review? The aim of this chapter is to discuss the practicalities involved in the day-to-day management of people with an LTC in primary care and encourage you to start thinking about the service you currently provide; how can you make it better?

PROTOCOLS

The words protocol, protocol-based care and protocol-based services feature in many of the UK guiding government policies, particularly in the National Service Frameworks (NSFs). Indeed, they were considered an integral part of the NHS plan (DoH 2000b, p. 83), which stated:

> By 2004 the majority of the NHS will be working under agreed protocols identifying how common conditions should be handled and which staff can best handle them. The new NHS Modernisation Agency will lead a major drive to ensure that protocol based care takes hold throughout the NHS. It will work with the National Institute for Clinical Excellence [NICE], patients, clinicians and managers to develop clear protocols that make the best use of all the talents of NHS staff and which are flexible enough to take account of patients' individual needs.

Protocols have long been used in the primary care setting to guide practice, define the roles of health care professionals and provide a guide to all those involved in the day-to-day practicalities of care provision. A protocol should:

• be an agreed strategy for carrying out a procedure or activity;
• be evidence-based but reflect local need;
• form a structured framework to prevent duplication of services and maintain standards among all team members;
• identify clear roles of responsibility for all those involved;
• be an integral part of the audit cycle evaluating patient care.

So what sorts of practical issues should be included in a protocol for people with LTCs? Table 7.1 provides a guide to the general areas that should be addressed within a protocol.

Table 7.1 Protocol

- Register – who maintains and updates it?
- Recall system – computer or paper based?
- Identification of a system to recall people who do not attend (DNA).
- General administration issues (who will be responsible for sending review/recall letters, what system will be put in place to ensure that they are informed if someone DNAs or cannott attend an appointment?).
- Timing of clinic/appointment (will it suit the client need – are this client group of working age, would an early morning/evening clinic appointment be more appropriate?).
- Timing of appointments (how long is required – need to consider newly diagnosed, routine review and annual review).
- Location.
- Resources required (for both clinical issues, e.g. Doppler for peripheral arterial diseae (PAD) assessment, tuning fork for diabetic foot assessment, spirometer for respiratory review and also supportive literature, e.g. peak flow/blood glucose-monitoring diaries, literature related to self-help groups, condition specific leaflets).
- How often should review take place (six monthly/annually)?
- What will be incorporated into the review (routine and annual)?
- Role of each health care professional, e.g. HCA (health care assistant), registered nurse, GP (general practitioner), dietician, podiatrist, pharmacist?
- Educational needs of each health care professional involved (e.g. if HCAs take blood pressure, who teaches them that skill? Would the clinic be improved if the registered nurse providing the care has an independent prescribing qualification, have GPs attended regular updates to ensure their knowledge is up to date regarding the LTCs they are responsible for?)
- Physical parameters to be measured: height/weight/body mass index (BMI)/blood tests/blood pressure/urinalysis.
- Which, if any, of these physical parameters need to be performed prior to the review appointment so that results are available at review?
- Type of physical/clinical examination to be performed and by whom?
- Medication review.
- Type of psychological assessment to be performed and by whom?
- Education: for both the person with the LTC, family and carers, what needs to be included, e.g. advice re driving, restricted occupations, self-care.
- Available local initiatives, e.g. expert patient programme.
- Referral criteria – both within and outside the team.
- Audit – how will the quality of the care provided be measured?
- Protocol review date – at least yearly, or earlier if new evidence dictates.

Developing a protocol

Developing a protocol should not be an individual activity. Although it is a good idea for one person to take overall responsibility for its production and regular review, the protocol should be written in discussion with all those who are going to be involved in the care, including administration staff who will be vital in ensuring that everything runs smoothly and efficiently. Discussion of the protocol should be considered as part of a team-building/educational exercise, using the opportunity to review everyone's role and to identify individual and/or group educational needs to ensure effective care delivery.

PAUSE FOR REFLECTION

Is everyone who is going to be involved in care delivery up to date with the latest research/clinical guidelines for the condition being discussed? Would any of the individuals providing care benefit from attending a specific structured education programme or would it be more beneficial to arrange in-house training led by a group member with expertise, or a local expert in the field?

With the increasing incidence of LTCs and the number of conditions classed as long term, some primary health care teams have moved away from running specific condition clinics (e.g. diabetes, asthma) and now include regular designated appointments for people with LTCs incorporated into their general clinics. This can often be beneficial for patients with LTCs as it removes the restriction of appointments always being on a specific day, which may be inconvenient. This type of system can work well, but administration procedures need to be highly efficient, especially if different health care professionals deal with particular specialities. All members of the primary health care team should be aware of the key principles involved in general management of people with an LTC, but for people requiring more specialist advice or treatment systems will need to be put into place to ensure that they are given an appointment with the most appropriate person. Appointment times will also need to be adjusted accordingly to ensure adequate time is made available for the review. When developing protocols, although broad principles such as registration and recall systems and appointment times may be similar for each LTC, a protocol will be required for each LTC to take into account condition-specific needs and treatment packages.

THE THREE RS: REGISTRATION/RECALL/REVIEW

Registration/recall

Throughout this book the importance of the three Rs has been clearly emphasised; if you don't know who your client group is, how can you meet their needs? The first key strand of the English *NHS Social Care Model to Support Local Innovation and Integration* (DoH 2005c), discussed in Chapter 1, is infrastructure. At the centre of the strand is decision support tools and clinical information systems (NpfIT) which, together with community resources and a health and social care system environment, support all aspects of the delivery system (case management, disease management, supported self-care and promoting better health), in turn creating better health outcomes. The model continues to outline IT systems that can support information sharing and the three Rs – registration, recall and review – as a fundamental feature of this strand, in addition to the Quality and Outcomes Framework (QOF), NICE and NSFs (see Chapter 1).

How to identify people who have an LTC and the criteria to firmly establish diagnosis has been discussed in the previous chapter. Once diagnosis has been confirmed, an initial appointment to develop an appropriate care plan and treatment package should be arranged and details of the LTC coded and entered on to a database. In the UK this will be within the GP practice. Since the implementation of the General Medical Services (GMS) contract (BMA/NHS Confederation 2003) and the QOF, information systems are in place within each GP practice in the UK to ensure that information regarding people with LTCs is regularly inputted and updated. The implementation of QOF has contributed greatly to the precision of data related to incidence and prevalence of LTCs through accurate registration. This also encourages practices to check their records for accuracy if these show that prevalence of a particular LTC is lower than would be normally expected within a similar patient population. However, as noted in Chapter 1, QOF is limited to specific LTCs and there is a danger that patients who have an LTC not covered by a QOF will not be included on a condition-specific register or be called for regular review. It is well established that ad hoc review (people making appointments when they feel they need to be seen) is not the most appropriate or effective system in providing care for people with LTCs and regular review systems should be put in place for all those with LTCs.

PAUSE FOR REFLECTION

If UK based, does your database only contain registers of people with LTCs covered by a QOF? Do you have a system in place to ensure regular review of people with LTCs not covered by a QOF (e.g. osteoporosis)?

If not UK based, what systems do you have in place to ensure adequate registration and recall of people with LTCs? Is this IT based or paper based and how well does it work – are people lost to recall?

Identifying people with an LTC involves clinicians searching for patients in their electronic records systems against a series of codes within the clinical system. There are many coding systems used in health care (within the UK: Read Codes, dm+d, OPCS and internationally ICD-10 and SNOME: see http://www.connectingforhealth.nhs.uk/systemsandservices/data/terminology).

Clinical systems all have search facilities, which allow for searches of electronic health records (EHRs) for particular codes. Most primary care system providers have reports embedded in their electronic clinical management systems that help with identifying patients with an LTC. These are based on code formulae (sometimes nationally agreed, e.g. QOF codes) that can find a patient who is likely to have an LTC identified in their EHR. A further way to identify patients is opportunistically. Most patients with an LTC will attend their practice several times a year (some several times a month) so that their records can be flagged with correct LTC codes. When a patient attends for the first time to register with a practice it is essential to record codes for his or her LTC.

When a patient is newly diagnosed and the practice receives information to this effect it is most important to correctly record this LTC code or codes into his or her EHR.

Those without the appropriate IT systems in place that provide automatic inclusion on the register once a correct read code is entered on the system can still identify patients through a number of methods. A search for a condition-specific heading or condition-specific drugs can help narrow the search. Records can then be cross-checked to ensure accurate classification. It is vital that all practitioners check that correct read codes are used to ensure that people with LTCs are identified by the system; regular educational updates should be arranged for all staff to prevent potential errors. Once an adequate registration system has been put in place, a recall procedure to ensure regular review needs to be developed. This can be achieved by implementation of a suitable IT programme that recalls people for review at a set time following their last appointment (e.g. six months or annually). Alternatively, a system can be adopted/developed that relates to annual recall through alphabetical order or month of birth. More frequent appointments can then be arranged as necessary, but the system will ensure that everyone is recalled at least annually. For example:

- All people with diabetes with a surname beginning with A or B are called for review in January, Cs and Ds in February, and so on.

Or

- All people with diabetes are called for review in the month of their birth: January, February, and so on.

Or

- The time for the next appointment can be decided at the visit and a recall system put in place whereby a recall letter is sent automatically two weeks before the due date.

Where adequate IT systems are not in place or a different type of system is preferred, the following are suitable options:

- The next appointment is booked at the current visit and an appointment card given. If this is more than six months in the future it is a good idea to follow it up with a reminder letter nearer the time.
- A card index (or diary) system can be utilised where, after each appointment, the person's details are placed in a filing system sorted by month. A recall letter is then sent out with an appointment date and time and, two weeks prior to the due date, to all people filed under that month. Although this is now considered a relatively old-fashioned method it would be an appropriate system in countries where IT support is limited.

People who are unable to attend or do not attend their appointment will need to be offered a rescheduled appointment. In addition, people who perhaps have received their review in secondary care will need to be advised that two review appointments are not necessary; a system of cross-checking can cancel recall letters for this small group. Housebound patients with LTCs have often been a neglected group in terms of regular review, and although the enhanced registration systems associated with QOF have led to improved systems, it is vital that each practice identifies who is going to take responsibility for reviewing housebound patients. These are often people who are not necessarily on the district nursing caseload; responsibility for delivery of the appropriate care package needs to be negotiated by the team.

Review

The majority of people with LTCs will need at minimum a full annual review carried out according to an appropriate evidence-based clinical guideline or current research recommendations. Each specific condition will have different requirements regarding physical parameters, clinical examination and treatment options; these should be based on appropriate evidence (see Chapter 8 for sources of evidence). Condition presentation, disease progression and co-morbidities must be taken into account; these will vary according to the individual. All people with LTCs will need education and discussion regarding the principles of self-management, supported with appropriate literature. These should be addressed at diagnosis and reinforced at each visit. Referral to local educational/self-management programmes should be made where available and dependent on the individual; as noted earlier, self-management programmes are not suitable for everyone. Following the first initial appointment after diagnosis, a care/treatment plan should be developed in conjunction with the health care professional, the person with the LTC and his or her family/carers as appropriate. Follow-up appointments will depend on individual need and should take into account the severity of the presenting condition, and educational, social and cultural needs. As noted in Chapter 4, the development of concordance is one of the key elements in developing a care plan that meets individual need but also maximises treatment options. Examples of a primary care annual review for a person with epilepsy (Table 7.2) and a person with diabetes (Table 7.3) are shown below. Please refer to an appropriate evidence-based guideline for further details and treatment options.

Table 7.4 includes general recommendations, taken from SIGN (2004) and CKS (2006c), relating to the types of issues that could be included in a review of a patient with osteoporosis. At the time of publication UK NICE guidelines were under review.

Table 7.2 Example of an annual structured review for an adult with epilepsy

- Information should be provided to the person with epilepsy and their family/carers.
- The following should be discussed: (1) seizure control; (2) any adverse effects of medication; (3) concordance with current medication.
- If seizure control is inadequate: (1) ensure medication is being taken correctly as prescribed; (2) specialist advice should be sought, or a referral made, before medication is changed; (3) epilepsy specialist nurses are good resources to discuss any issues identified within the review.
- It should be ascertained that all people with epilepsy have (1) an accessible point of contact with specialist services; (2) a comprehensive care plan in place; (3) access to an epilepsy specialist nurse.
- Regular blood test monitoring is not recommended unless clinically indicated (e.g. suspected toxicity, adjustment of phenytoin dose).
- Blood tests for full blood count (fbc), electrolytes, liver enzymes, vitamin D and other tests of bone metabolism should be performed two to five times yearly in adults taking enzyme-inducing drugs.

(adapted from CKS 2006b)

Table 7.3 Example of an annual structured review for an adult with type 2 diabetes

- At least one week prior to review (to ensure results are available for discussion at review): HbA1c (glycated haemoglobin), urea and electrolytes (including serum creatinine), estimated glomerular filtration rate (eGFR), liver function tests, full lipid screen, thyroid function tests, early morning urine for albumin/creatinine (ACR) ratio (in the absence of proteinurea/urinary tract infection);
- blood pressure;
- BMI/waist measurement;
- examination of patient's feet and lower legs to detect risk factors, including: testing of foot sensation using 10g microfilament or vibration, palpation of foot pulses, inspection for foot deformity, inspection of footwear; management plan agreed including foot care education, or referral if indicated by assessment.
- questions asked about neuropathic symptoms (e.g. foot problems, erectile dysfunction, gastroparesis);
- individual ongoing nutritional advice given by a health care professional with specific expertise;
- discussion of self-monitoring of blood glucose, where appropriate;
- ongoing structured patient education offered to the person with diabetes, his or her family and carers;
- discussion of lifestyle issues (e.g. smoking cessation, exercise);
- structured screening for depression;
- monitoring of structured eye surveillance has been performed (ideally through quality assured retinal photography programme);
- cardiovascular risk review;
- medication review.

(adapted from NICE 2008)

Table 7.4 Potential areas to include in a review of a patient with osteoporosis

---

- Education regarding disease process and importance of intervention therapies.
- Medication review – concordance with current therapy/review of any side effects.
- Pain assessment.
- Any falls since last review?
- Discussion (to include family/carers as appropriate) re interventions to prevent falls; i.e. modifying home environment, modifying living habits (such as wearing of appropriate footwear), installing appropriate aids (handrails, non slip bathmat), modifying medications that may predispose to falls, correction of poor vision, referral to appropriate support services.
- Discussion re lifestyle factors (e.g. weight, smoking, alcohol consumption).
- Advice re exercise programmes including high-intensity strength training and low-impact weight bearing exercise.
- If repeat dual-energy x-ray absorptiometry (DXA) scanning is thought to be appropriate, in general this should not be carried out unless the person has been taking treatment for at least two years.
- Repeat DXA scanning should be considered if a woman has another fragility fracture despite adhering fully to treatment with a bisphosphonate for first year.

(CKS 2006c)

Evidence supporting the three Rs

The benefits of organisational interventions to improve recall and review, in addition to multifaceted interventions to improve the performance of practitioners in enhancing the care of people with diabetes, have been demonstrated in two Cochrane systematic reviews (Griffin and Kinmonth 2000; Renders *et al.* 2001). This was further supported by a large randomised controlled trial (RCT) in Denmark (Olivarius *et al.* 2001) that randomised general practitioners to a control and intervention group. The intervention group were given patient leaflets, guidelines, annual seminars and feedback, prompted to review patients, encouraged to set and subsequently revise realistic treatment goals and were exposed to a charismatic opinion leader. Additional interventions to improve care of diabetes in the community included patient education and support for self-management, changes in delivery systems such as enhancement of the involvement of nurses, and additional decision support for practitioners. Results indicated statistically significant improvements in both glycated haemoglobin and BP, with subsequent observed risk reductions in cardiovascular and microvascular complications. Griffin (2001) noted that caution should be taken in interpreting the results, in that the recruited GPs were particularly motivated, further noting that many primary care teams outside these research studies fail to achieve the same intensive management of multiple risk factors. He emphasises the question: once the three Rs are firmly established what is it that makes the difference? Was it the setting and reassessment of personalised, realistic goals by practitioners, congruent with evidence from psychology, or that patients who received the intervention are more actively involved in their care, more satisfied, and more likely to adhere to medication than those in routine care? Whatever the reasons behind the improved health outcomes, it is important that practitioners take the message from studies such as these on board and review the way they provide care to maximise overall health outcomes for all people with LTCs.

Fahey *et al.* (2006) conducted a Cochrane systematic review relating to people with hypertension with two key objectives:

- to determine the effectiveness of interventions to improve control of blood pressure in patients with hypertension;
- to evaluate the effectiveness of reminders on improving the follow-up of patients with hypertension.

Similar results were seen as in previous reviews. Fifty-six RCTs met the inclusion criteria, six types of interventions were reviewed including: self-monitoring, educational interventions directed to the patient, educational interventions directed to the health professional, health professional (nurse or pharmacist)-led care, organisational interventions that aimed to improve the delivery of care, and appointment reminder systems. Results did vary according to each intervention. Self-monitoring was associated with moderate net reduction in diastolic blood pressure and appointment reminders increased the proportion of individuals who attended for follow-up. Educational interventions directed at patients or health professionals, however, appeared unlikely to be associated with large net reductions in blood pressure. Health professional (nurse or pharmacist)-led care appeared to be a promising way of delivering care but requires further evaluation. Fahey *et al.* (2006) concluded that despite the variability of methodological quality and the heterogenous results from RCTs related to some of the interventions, an organised system of regular follow-up and review, combined with a vigorous stepped care approach to antihypertensive drug treatment, appeared to be the most likely way to improve the control of high blood pressure.

In relation to epilepsy, Redhead (2003) noted that despite epilepsy being the most common serious neurological disorder in the UK, a lack of neurologists means that patients' day-to-day prescribing, supervision and support often depend on primary care. He suggested that an improvement in the process of care in the primary care setting can result from three important strategies:

> appropriately trained practice nurses running practice nurse-led clinics; structured management of care, through registration, which facilitates audit, prescription monitoring, and recall; and, finally, improved teamwork and communication based on protocols locally agreed upon between primary and secondary care.
>
> (Redhead 2003, p. 54)

There is clear evidence that structured programmes of care with efficient registration and recall systems have a positive effect on health outcomes and in most areas there is always room for improvement. This was clearly demonstrated in the Improvement Foundation's National Primary Care Collaborative Programme which, prior to the implementation of the new GMS (nGMS) contract (BMA/NHS Confederation 2003), set up a programme to help GP practices achieve improvements for patients with established cardiovascular disease – secondary prevention. Later phases of the programme included diabetes and chronic obstructive pulmonary disease (COPD). The aim of the work was to ensure that patients received optimum care through the application of a systematic, sustainable approach. The benefits demonstrated by the programme in improving the management of LTCs were later incorporated into a QOF. The programme worked with practices, asking them to focus their efforts around a number of key principles; these were:

- Know all your patients who have CHD [coronary heart disease]
- Be systematic and proactive in managing care
- Ensure timely and high-quality support from secondary care
- Involve patients in delivering and developing care
- Develop effective links with other key local partners.
  (Improvement Foundation 2008)

Case studies demonstrating how practices improved their care are available on the Improvement Foundation website. These included developing practice agreed protocols, telephone reminders to non-attenders, sending practice nurses on a validated training programme to enable them to run enhanced CHD clinics and holding educational events for GPs run by the local cardiologist, among other initiatives. Overall results of the CHD secondary prevention programme, which included a total of 5,442 general practices, indicated a fourfold reduction in mortality for patients with CHD in participating Primary Care Trusts compared to non-participants. This was equivalent to 3,000 lives from myocardial infarctions (MIs) saved per year and a reduction of non-fatal MIs by 3,000 per year. The Improvement Foundation states that it has improved the care of LTCs across thousands of practices in England, Scotland, Canada and Australia. Information on its latest programmes is available at: http://www.improvementfoundation.org/theme/long-term-conditions.

TEAMWORK AND REFERRAL CRITERIA

As teams develop and skill mix in health care delivery becomes a more popular concept in primary care the importance of referral criteria and a clear awareness of each other's roles becomes even more important. The benefits of a multi-disciplinary approach and the importance of teamwork have been discussed in Chapter 3, but within the primary health care setting an awareness of the roles of all those involved, including the patient and carer, is essential. A team approach to care can improve accessibility for people with LTCs and expand the range of services offered. Clear referral criteria should, however, be built into the protocol to ensure that each team member is aware of his or her limitations and is aware of when it is appropriate to seek more specialised advice. Clear channels of communication should be established and maintained to ensure that people referred to other members of the team are seen quickly and by the most appropriate person.

AUDIT

How the service provided will be monitored and evaluated should be an integral part of protocol development, through the process of clinical audit. Clinical audit has been defined as:

> the systematic and critical analysis of the quality of clinical care, a quality improvement process that seeks to improve patient care and outcomes through systematic review of care against explicit criteria and the implementation of change.
>
> (NICE 2002)

Clinical audit is a central feature of the clinical governance umbrella, the organisational approach to quality introduced in the UK as a response to concerns about quality of health care in the NHS, most notably the Bristol inquiry, a public inquiry into children's heart surgery in the Bristol Royal Infirmary from 1984 to 1995. Clinical governance was defined in the DoH (1998) consultation document *A First Class Service: Quality in the New NHS* as:

> a framework through which NHS organisations are accountable for continuously improving the quality of their services and safeguarding high standards of care by creating an environment in which excellence in clinical care will flourish.

The clinical governance umbrella consists of a number of key components, including:

- patient, public and carer involvement;
- risk management – Incident reporting, infection control, prevention and control of risk;
- staff management and performance – recruitment, workforce planning, appraisals;
- education, training and continuous professional development;
- clinical audit management, planning and monitoring, learning through research and audit;
- information management;

- communication – patient and public, external partners, internal, board and organisation-wide;
- leadership;
- teamworking.

The aim of clinical audit is to: assess and improve quality of care, act as an aid to continuing professional development, provide individuals and teams with a sense of both personal and professional achievement and to assess what one is doing and whether one can make it better. One of the recommendations of the Bristol inquiry was that clinical audit should be at the core of a system of local monitoring of performance and should be compulsory for all health care professionals providing clinical care. When conducted well, clinical audit provides a way in which quality of care can be reviewed objectively within a supportive and developmental culture. Audit has a number of well-documented key features that clearly distinguish it from research which have been reproduced in a number of audit training manuals; these are outlined in Table 7.5.

Clinical audit is about getting it right, ensuring the service you provide is evidence-based and effective and meets the needs of the people at whom it is aimed. Since the introduction of QOF many of the clinical targets relating to LTCs are included in a regular audit programme; for example:

- The percentage of patients on the diabetes register who have an HbA1c is recorded.
- The percentage of patients on the chronic kidney disease (CKD) register with hypertension and proteinuria who are treated with an angiotensin-converting enzyme inhibitor (ACE) or angiotensin receptor blocker (ARB) is recorded.

However, audit should also include quality issues such as people's perceptions of the type of service offered and whether it meets their needs. The key stages of audit include:

- Select a topic.
- Decide on element of care or activity to be measured – criteria (e.g. HbA1c).
- Set an appropriate and realistic standard (e.g. 85 per cent of all people on diabetes register).

Table 7.5 Research/audit

Research	Audit
Discovers the right thing to do	Determines whether the right thing is being done
A series of 'one-off' projects	A cyclical series of reviews
Collects complex data	Collects routine data
Experiment rigorously defined	Review of what clinicians actually do
Often possible to generalise the findings	Not possible to generalise from the findings

- Collect data.
- Evaluate findings, assess performance against criteria and standard.
- Act to make improvements, making any relevant changes identified as required.
- Repeat data collection and evaluation and take further action if required.

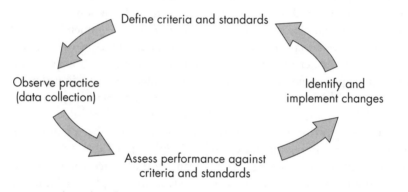

Figure 7.1 The audit cycle

CONCLUSION

This chapter has addressed many of the practical issues relating to providing systematic and structured care to people with LTCs in the primary care environment. It is recommended that primary health care teams review the services they provide and ensure that systems are in place to review all patients with an LTC, incorporating both generic principles of care and condition-specific elements. Regardless of the type of LTC, structured protocols, developed by all the team members who are to be involved in the care provision, should be developed and regularly updated, either annually or as new evidence dictates. Audit criteria should be built into the protocol to ensure that the service provided meets the needs of people with LTCs.

KEY POINTS

- Structured organisational interventions such as regular follow-up and review and appointment reminders improve overall health outcomes for people with LTCs.
- Regularly updated protocols may be used as a team-building exercise and also to identify educational needs of team members.

- Clinical audit criteria and standards should be considered as an integral part of protocol development.

FURTHER AREAS TO CONSIDER

- Are structured protocols in place for LTCs in your practice area, and do they address all conditions?
- Do you meet regularly as a team to discuss new evidence that may have an impact on effective health care delivery?
- Who is responsible for ensuring that local protocols are updated and reflect recent evidence?
- Does each team member understand the others' roles and when it is appropriate to refer to another team member?

CHAPTER 8

EVIDENCE-BASED PRACTICE

OVERVIEW

What do we mean by evidence-based practice (EBP)? How does one access appropriate evidence? This chapter provides a definition and brief history, followed by a guide to how to formulate a question and search for appropriate evidence. This includes a guide to evidence-based clinical guidelines relating to long-term conditions (LTCs), including appropriate website addresses.

INTRODUCTION

Previous chapters have demonstrated the numerous and differing types and varieties of conditions that may be classed as LTCs. Diagnostic criteria have been discussed relating to some of these conditions, as well as the general principles regarding care of people with LTCs. It is not, however, within the scope of this book to provide specific management advice and guidance for every type of LTC. The aim of this chapter then is to discuss the principles of evidence-based practice, including definition and brief historical development, along with a guide to relevant websites and evidence-based clinical guidelines to ensure that the reader is aware of how and where to access condition-specific evidence-based information. The difference between primary and secondary (evaluated) sources of information will be introduced as well as guidance on how to answer a clinical question, including phrasing the question, developing a search strategy and critical appraisal.

DEFINITIONS AND BRIEF HISTORY OF EVIDENCE-BASED PRACTICE

EBP has been at the forefront of effective health care for some time. The foundations of today's EBP originally lay in evidence-based medicine (EBM), whose philosophical origins date back to nineteenth-century Paris. The introduction of evidence-based medicine and its effect on changing medical practice has been described as a paradigm shift, largely attributed to developments in clinical research. The EBM movement has expanded rapidly since the 1990s and now includes all aspects of health care. Indeed, within the UK the aim of the national research and development programme launched by the NHS back in 1991 (DoH 1991) was to close the gap between health care demonstrated to be effective through research and the health care actually delivered. Since this time EBP has continued to move on with increasing speed and vigour. The aim of EBP today is to ensure that all health care practice is firmly grounded in a sound evidence base that also takes into account individual patient needs and preferences. Sackett *et al.*'s (1996, p. 71) classic definition of evidence-based medicine states that:

> Evidence based medicine is the conscientious, explicit, and judicious use of current best evidence in making decisions about the care of individual patients. The practice of evidence based medicine means integrating individual clinical expertise with the best available external clinical evidence from systematic research.

Others have since expanded upon this definition to signify the importance of EBP to all health care professionals and to further emphasise the importance of taking into account individual patient/client needs and preferences when considering appropriate evidence. The Joanna Briggs Institute (JBI), an international collaboration providing evidence-based health care resources, defines evidence-based practice as:

> The melding of individual clinical judgement and expertise with the best available external evidence to generate the kind of practice that is most likely to lead to a positive outcome for a client or patient.

The Institute further provides a definition of evidence-based nursing as:

> Nursing practice that is characterised by these attributes. Evidence based clinical practice takes into account the context within which

care takes place; the preferences of the client; and the clinical judgement of the health professional, as well as the best available evidence.

Initiatives to improve access to research findings have developed rapidly over the past 15 to 20 years as a result of the international commitment to evidence-based health care. The Cochrane Collaboration, first launched in 1993, and named after the British epidemiologist Archie Cochrane, has played a leading role in developing and promoting evidence-based health care and continues to be one of the finest resources in developing methodology related to systematic reviews of health care interventions. Back in the 1970s Archie Cochrane suggested that the most effective use of limited heath care resources would be to equitably provide health care interventions that had been shown to be effective. In addition to stressing the importance of utilising evidence from randomised controlled trials (RCTs), he challenged both his profession and the establishment to produce regularly updated critical summaries of all RCTs. His encouragement, supported by others in his profession, led to the establishment of the Cochrane Collaboration (http://www.cochrane.org/docs/archieco.htm).

The principles of EBP were developed in the Department of Clinical Epidemiology and Biostatistics at McMasters University in Canada in the 1980s, where a group of practitioners wanted to find new ways of finding, appraising and using research, and to develop systematic and scientific principles to help clinicians make decisions based on the best information available. Within the UK centres for EBP developed rapidly, supported by modern disciples such as David Sackett and colleagues. Sackett *et al.*'s BMJ (1996) editorial 'Evidence based medicine: what it is and what it isn't' is fundamental reading for those interested in EBP.

In addition to EBP centres and collaborations providing systematic reviews, a surfeit of evidence-based journals and increasing numbers of evidence-based clinical guidelines and critical reviews are now available. The more these sources become available, however, the more confusion is created for practitioners who need to be sure that the evidence they are accessing is up to date and relevant to their practice. A guide to some of these will be provided later in the chapter, but first some of the principles and steps involved in EBP will be discussed.

APPLYING EVIDENCE TO PRACTICE

A number of steps are involved in applying an evidence-based approach to practice. According to Cullum (2000), these include:

- Reflecting on practice to identify areas of uncertainty.
- Translating areas of uncertainty into focused, searchable questions.
- Searching the literature for appropriate studies that answer the question.

- Critically appraising the research.
- Changing practice, if the research findings suggest that is necessary, and evaluating the changes.

Reflection

The first step in applying evidence to practice is to recognise that there may be a gap between current practice and the best evidence for what constitutes effective practice. The NHS Executive (1999) uses the term 'unsubstantiated certainty' to refer to the certainty practitioners have that a particular approach which is not based on reliable evidence is correct. Practitioners should continually question and reflect on their current practice and be aware of clues that indicate best practice has moved on. Greenhalgh (2001) notes that although we may think EBP is something we have always done, estimates in the 1980s suggested that only about 10 to 20 per cent of medical interventions were evidence-based; although these figures were later disputed, a further evaluation classified 21 per cent of health technologies as evidence-based.

PAUSE FOR REFLECTION

Have you ever practised with 'unsubstantiated certainty'? Do you know what the evidence base is for all the procedures you carry out?

Formulating a question

The second step is to formulate an appropriate question from an initial concern or 'woolly thoughts'. This process will help define exactly what you need to know. You may have a large knowledge base on a particular topic, but how do you translate this into a succinct summary of the problem that includes any additional information you may need to solve it (Greenhalgh 2001)? A number of authors have proposed suitable methodologies to assist in formulating the problem in order to search the literature for the appropriate evidence (Flemming 1998; Sackett et al. 2000). All suggest that a well-built question should have three or four elements. For example, in the 'PICO' method, recommended by the NHS Executive (1999), the key elements are:

- Problem
- Intervention
- Comparison
- Outcome.

Table 8.1 The PICO method

What is the best method of helping people diagnosed with asthma to recognise the signs of an asthma exacerbation?

Problem: In adults diagnosed with asthma.

Intervention: What are the benefits of teaching regular peak flow measurement?

Comparison: Instead of, or in addition to, teaching recognition of deteriorating asthma through identification of specific symptoms.

Outcome: In reducing the overall incidence of emergency consultations/admissions for asthma exacerbation.

The focus of the question may be diagnosis, prognosis, a health care intervention, or the cost-effectiveness or efficiency of an intervention (NHS Executive 1999). The PICO method may be used to translate initial thoughts about a gap between evidence and practice into an answerable question. For example, a question such as 'What is the best method of helping people diagnosed with asthma to recognise the signs of an asthma exacerbation?' could be translated into four parts using the PICO method (Table 8.1). Framing the question in this way not only makes it possible to think harder about the individual aspects of the problem, and what you actually need to know, but also helps define the search terms, which is important for database searching.

Not all questions will relate to research studies that use quantitative methods. For example, a question such as 'What methods do people diagnosed with asthma feel are the most helpful for recognising early signs of an asthma exacerbation?' would be better answered by studies utilising qualitative methods of inquiry. To answer questions that involve finding out the person's or carer's viewpoint on a particular intervention, or to gain understanding about a condition from their perspective, the PICO method can still be used or a different acronym may be useful for answering the question. The SPICE acronym (Table 8.2) includes the following elements:

- Setting
- Perspective
- Intervention or interpretation
- Comparison
- Evaluation.

PAUSE FOR REFLECTION

Think of a problem you have come across relating to LTC management, where you were not sure of the evidence base, and express it as an answerable question using the PICO or SPICE method.

Table 8.2 The SPICE acronym

What methods do people diagnosed with asthma feel are the most helpful for recognising early signs of an asthma exacerbation?

Setting: In adults diagnosed with asthma in the primary care setting.

Perspective: What are their feelings?

Intervention: About the usefulness of written treatment plans.

Comparison: Instead of, or in addition to, teaching recognition of deteriorating asthma through identification of specific symptoms?

Evaluation: relating to increased self-confidence in recognising early asthma exacerbation and instigating treatment.

Searching for evidence

The third step, searching for the evidence, is one that nurses and other health care professionals often find the most difficult. A search of large databases such as CINAHL (Current Index to Nursing and Allied Health Literature) or PubMed (publicly available MEDLINE) can be time consuming and frustrating for inexperienced users, who, because of a lack of knowledge of advanced searching techniques, may either find vast amounts of inappropriate information or, alternatively, may miss essential information. For a busy nurse working in primary care who needs to find information quickly, such databases may appear daunting.

PAUSE FOR REFLECTION

Are you skilled in database searching or have you ever experienced frustration when trying to find an answer? Think about what databases you have accessed and whether you have had any difficulties with searching: do you find too much or too little information? Have you had instruction in database searching or accessed online tutorials?

Critical appraisal

Once the evidence has been found, the fourth step is critical appraisal, which can also prove difficult for those with limited time. Fortunately, there are easy ways to access information that has been subjected to a variety of forms of critical review. A question may already have been asked and the answer may be available in a critically appraised study, but the key is in knowing where to look. The first thing to know is that research exists in two forms: primary evidence (e.g. RCTs, cohort studies, case control studies, qualitative studies) and evaluated or secondary resources (systematic reviews, meta-analyses, clinical guidelines, narrative or meta-synthesis, critical reviews, query-answering services) (Bidwell 2004). It can be time consuming to sift through primary evidence and sometimes studies can be contradictory; or more accessible research reports can exaggerate the effects of interventions. Secondary sources aim to track down all information, including that which may be inaccessible to practitioners. This information is then appraised using robust methods.

Systematic reviews and meta-analyses are considered the 'gold standard' of evidence for quantitative (positivist) research, because they use explicit criteria to identify and appraise all the literature on a particular topic (NHS Executive 1999). Systematic reviews of evidence favour meta-analysis of RCTs, considered 'gold standard' in trials of effectiveness (cause and effect), with other quantitative methods ranked lower in terms of effectiveness. Narrative synthesis and meta-synthesis have more recently been developed as methods to combine findings from qualitative (naturalistic) research, mixed methods studies, or quantitative studies where a statistical approach to combining findings is not necessarily the best method (Centre for Reviews and Dissemination (CRD) 2005; JBI 2008). These methods appreciate that while RCTs are the best methods for answering 'cause-and-effect' questions, interpretive and qualitative research methods are more appropriate in studies aimed at exploring and interpreting experiences and gaining a more in-depth understanding of human behaviour.

Good-quality guidelines and critical reviews will have used a comprehensive search strategy to track down all the evidence on a specific topic and will have used a robust critical appraisal tool to determine their overall findings and recommendations. High-calibre guidelines should provide advice to practitioners based on the best evidence available and will utilise systematic reviews, where accessible, to develop these recommendations. Critical reviews can vary in quality, depending on the search strategy utilised, and can be biased towards the author's opinion if limited literature is accessed. A third source of evidence is query-answering services, which provide a valuable service to busy practitioners. They conduct 'quick and dirty' searches, which although not of the same standard as systematic reviews, utilise established quality criteria and point practitioners in the right direction of available evidence. They too utilise systematic reviews and high-calibre guidelines, where available, to provide an answer, but will also provide brief critical appraisals and summaries of other sources of evidence in areas where less substantial bodies of evidence are obtainable.

For those wishing to learn more about critical appraisal, Trisha Greenhalgh's (2001) book *How to Read a Paper* is essential reading. In addition to this there are many organisations that provide training in critical skills appraisal such as the Critical Appraisal Skills Programme (CASP) that provides workshops and learning resources including appraisal tools to supply individuals and organisations with the skills to base not only their clinical practice, but also policy- and decision-making, on robust evidence of effectiveness.

PAUSE FOR REFLECTION

Have you ever changed your practice based on a headline-hitting article that you found when browsing through the latest clinical journals, or do you always seek out further supportive information before altering your practice?

FINDING RELIABLE SECONDARY (EVALUATED) SOURCES

UK portals

A number of sites provide access to evaluated high-quality information. Accessing these sites first can reduce searching time and also ensure that the information found is both of high quality and has been subjected to regular updating in light of new evidence. Within the UK NHS websites provide free and easy access to evidence-based sites that were previously restricted to subscribers (Table 8.3). All NHS staff, or those caring for NHS patients, are able to apply for a password which allows access to numerous sites otherwise limited to subscribers. Details may be found in the NLH (England), Howis e-library (Wales), NHS Scotland, or HONNI (Northern Ireland).

ACCESSING SYSTEMATIC REVIEWS, META-ANALYSIS AND NARRATIVE SYNTHESIS

One of the best-known sources of both primary and secondary (evaluated) evidence is the Cochrane Library, which consists of a collection of regularly updated databases of evidence. A number of countries provide free access to the Cochrane Library for health care professionals through funded provision, including: all countries of the UK, Australia, New Zealand, Ireland, Finland, Poland, Norway, Sweden, India, parts of Canada, Wyoming in the USA, Latin America and the Caribbean, sponsored South African residents and low-income countries (please access Cochrane website for further details).

Table 8.3 UK NHS websites

National Library of Health (NLH) (England)	www.nelh.nhs.uk
HOWIS e-library (Wales)	www.wales.nhs.uk/sites3/home.cfm?orgid=520
HONNI (Northern Ireland)	www.honni.qub.ac.uk
NHS Scotland e-library	www.elib.scot.nhs.uk/portal/elib/pages/index.aspx

Table 8.4 Databases

The Cochrane Database of Systematic Reviews
Systematic reviews undertaken by the Cochrane Collaboration subject to specific evaluation criteria

The Database of Abstracts of Reviews of Effects (DARE)
A database maintained and created by the Centre for Reviews and Dissemination at the University of York (CRD): structured abstracts written by CRD reviewers of systematic reviews about the effects of interventions. Inclusion is subject to strict CRD quality criteria

Cochrane Methodology Register (CMR; Methods Studies)
A bibliography of publications which report on methods used in the conduct of controlled trials

Cochrane Central Register of Controlled Trials
A comprehensive collection of primary research studies

The Health Technology Assessment (HTA)
An excellent source of critical reviews

NHS Economic Evaluation Database (NHS EED)
A collection of economic evaluations

It is considered to be the first resource for information about the effects of health care interventions. It includes the DARE, HTA and NHS EED databases which can also be accessed directly from the website of the CRD at the University of York (Table 8.4).

CRD also provides a range of other services including an enquiry service that searches its databases for an answer to a question, and a helpdesk for searching the databases and information resources page. Other key sources of systematic reviews include the Berkeley Systematic Review Group in the USA and the aforementioned Australia-based Joanna Briggs Institute (Table 8.5). JBI includes four key aspects in its Model of Evidence-based Health Care: evidence generation, evidence synthesis, evidence transfer and evidence utilisation. In addition to considering international evidence related to the feasibility, appropriateness, meaningfulness and effectiveness of health care interventions and incorporating this evidence into systematic reviews, JBI globally disseminates information in the form of its *Best Practice Information* summary sheets. JBI also designs programs to enable the effective implementation of evidence and evaluation of its impact on health care practice.

Table 8.5 Sources of systematic reviews

Berkeley Systematic Reviews Group	http://www.medepi.org/meta/index.html
Centre for Reviews and Dissemination	http://www.york.ac.uk/inst/crd/
The Cochrane Library	www3.interscience.wiley.com/cgi-bin/mrwhome/ 106568753/HOME
The Joanna Briggs Institute	http://www.joannabriggs.edu.au/about/about.php

CLINICAL GUIDELINES

At one time clinical guidelines used to be an area of contention. A quick search of the worldwide web used to identify many that were not necessarily evidence-based. However, a number of established guideline sites now provide access to clear, evidence-based guidance developed according to stringent criteria. Indeed, there is even a research programme dedicated to 'reviewing the review' process. The Appraisal of Guidelines Research and Evaluation (AGREE), an international collaboration of researchers and policy-makers, has developed the AGREE instrument, a systematic framework to enable assessment of key components of guideline quality and to assist in the creation of a coordinated international approach to guideline development. Guidelines tend to provide advice relating to all aspects of specific conditions, particularly LTCs (unlike systematic reviews which tend to concentrate on one aspect of an intervention), and so are particularly useful to practitioners.

A number of UK organisations provide evidence-based guidelines on a range of clinical conditions including the Scottish Intercollegiate Guidelines Network (SIGN), the National Collaborating Centre for Chronic Conditions and the National Institute for Health and Clinical Excellence (NICE). The NLH Specialist Library guidelines finder is an easy way to find and access a wide range of evidence-based guidelines. Links are provided which are divided into condition-specific health problems, then further broken down into categories such as: diagnosis, causes and risk factors, prevention and disease management. Other organisations provide guidelines on particular conditions, e.g. the British Thoracic Society (BTS) and the British Hypertension Society (BHS). In addition to UK sites, there are some excellent international sites such as the Joanna Briggs Institute, US National Guideline Clearinghouse, the Australian National Health and Medical Research Council (NHMRC) Clinical Practice Guidelines and the New Zealand Guidelines Group, to name but a few.

PAUSE FOR REFLECTION

Are you aware of the latest evidence-based guidelines for all the types of LTCs that you manage? Does someone in your organisation take responsibility for disseminating the latest evidence?

OTHER GUIDELINE-RELATED RESOURCES

Clinical Evidence

Clinical Evidence is published by the BMJ Publishing Group. Currently online access is free for anyone accessing the site from Wales and Scotland through HOWIS or NHS Scotland e-library and for those accessing from a developing country, as part of the HINARI (Health InterNetwork Access to Research Initiative) which defines eligible countries; for further details see: http://clinical evidence.bmj.com/ceweb/about/onlineaccess_dev.jsp. It is also available via subscription, online, in print and through a personal digital assistant (PDA). The aim of *Clinical Evidence* is to cover a range of common or important clinical conditions seen in primary and hospital care. When deciding which conditions to cover, it reviews national data on consultation rates, morbidity and mortality, taking into account national priorities for health care such as those outlined in the UK National Service Frameworks and in the US Institute of Medicine reports, and also seeks the advice of generalist clinicians and patient groups. The questions in *Clinical Evidence* relate to the benefits and harms of preventive and therapeutic interventions, with an emphasis on outcomes that matter to patients (BMJ Clinical Evidence 2008).

Clinical Evidence uses a comprehensive search and appraisal strategy to summarise the most recent state of knowledge and uncertainty about the prevention and treatment of clinical conditions. To achieve this, for each of their systematic reviews they search the literature for other published systematic reviews and randomised controlled trials which answer the clinical questions, including EBM resources, major guideline sites such as NICE, and databases including Medline, EMBASE (Excerpta Medica Database) and the Cochrane Library. Where few or no good systematic reviews or randomised controlled trials are located it may also search for observational studies. *Clinical Evidence* currently provides evidence-based reviews of 2,500 treatments for over 250 conditions. If no good evidence is available, it says so. In addition, where good evidence is not available, it summarises guidelines and provides expert commentary, which is clearly distinguished from other usual evidence-based content. BMJ *Clinical Evidence* (2008) notes that although its intention was never to make recommendations, feeling that evidence should be individually interpreted, it has recently revisited this view, appreciating the frustration of practitioners who ask a question, only to be told that there is no evidence. To this end where evidence is weak, the site now also includes a 'comment' section to sum up what is available. Answers are provided in six clear categories to support individual practitioners in evidence-based decision-making:

- beneficial
- likely to be beneficial
- trade-off between benefits and harms

- unknown effectiveness
- unlikely to be beneficial
- likely to be ineffective or harmful.

Clinical Knowledge Summaries (CKS)

Probably one of the best sites in the UK providing clear and explicit guidelines for primary care is the NHS CKS site. This service is available free online to UK users. CKS's home page states that Clinical Knowledge Summaries are 'a reliable source of evidence-based information and practical 'know how' about the common conditions managed in primary care'. Information is presented in the form of clinical topics providing both quick and detailed answers to common questions that arise in consultations, relating to conditions seen regularly in primary care. In addition, CKS supplies a comprehensive range of well-written patient leaflets covering a wide range of conditions, that can be downloaded and given directly to the patient, as well as a Knowledge Plus section providing interesting knowledge and facts from credible, reliable sources.

TRIP (Turning Research Into Practice)

Two other excellent sources of evaluated research are the TRIP database and *Bandolier*. The TRIP database is now available free. Once a search term is entered, TRIP searches a range of evidence- based sites (e.g. *Clinical Evidence*, CKS, NICE, *Bandolier*) and simultaneously runs a PubMed search. This is much easier than making a separate search of each of these databases. Search results are automatically sorted into categories which include: evidence-based records, clinical guidelines, clinical questions and answers, eTextbook articles, medical images, patient leaflets and peer-reviewed journal articles. TRIP also has a 'specialist sites' collection; selecting 'Diabetes', for example, will search not only the core TRIP content but also eight of the leading diabetes journals. Users can also register to receive regular updates on topics of interest.

Bandolier

Bandolier is an independent evidence-based UK health care journal, written by Oxford scientists, available worldwide in print by annual subscription or free online. A print version of the journal is currently distributed to every GP in New Zealand. *Bandolier* finds information about effectiveness (or lack of it) through searching PubMed and the Cochrane Library, and reproduces the results from interesting systematic reviews and high-quality research in a simple format. *Bandolier* appears monthly and is an excellent source of evidence-based health care information provided in a well-written, straightforward and acerbic format, which is interesting and easy to read. In addition to the journal, *Bandolier* provides a range of other services that are worth a visit, including a Knowledge Library, Healthy Living zone, and the Oxford Pain internet site.

Query-answering services

There are two main question-answering services for primary care practitioners in the UK. The oldest is ATTRACT, which has been running since 1997 and is based in Wales. The other, started in 2004, is the NLH Primary Care Q&A Service. Although the NLH Q&A Service has now been discontinued while the commissioners undertake formal procurement, it is worthwhile accessing the NLH to review future services. Both services are similar in that members of the primary care team can leave a question on their websites. Teams of skilled information specialists undertake the hard work of locating the evidence and answering the question.

Clinical guidelines and related resources

AGREE

(Appraisal of Guidelines, Research and Evaluation) www.agreecollaboration. org/

ATTRACT

www.attract.wales.nhs.uk

Bandolier

www.jr2.ox.ac.uk/bandolier/

British Hypertension Society

http://www.bhsoc.org/Latest_BHS_management_Guidelines.stm

British Thoracic Society

www.brit-thoracic.org.uk

Critical Appraisal Skills Programme (CASP)

www.phru.nhs.uk/casp/casp.htm

Clinical Evidence

http://clinicalevidence.bmj.com/ceweb/index.jsp

Clinical Knowledge Summaries (CKS)

http://cks.library.nhs.uk/home

National Collaborating Centre for Chronic Conditions

http://www.rcplondon.ac.uk/clinical-standards/ncc-cc/Pages/NCC-CC.aspx

National Guideline Clearinghouse

www.guideline.gov/resources/guideline_index.aspx

National Health and Medical Research Council (NHMRC) Clinical Practice Guidelines

http://www.nhmrc.gov.au/publications/subjects/clinical.htm

National Institute for Health and Clinical Excellence (NICE)

www.nice.org.uk

National Library for Health (NLH)

www.nelh.nhs.uk

PubMed

www.ncbi.nlm.nih.gov/entrez/query.fcgi

School of Health and Related Research (ScHARR)

www.shef.ac.uk/scharr/ir/netting

Scottish Intercollegiate Guidelines Network (SIGN)

www.sign.ac.uk

TRIP

www.tripdatabase.com

New Zealand Guidelines Group

www.nzgg.org.nz/index.cfm?screensize=800&

CONCLUSION

A search of the above resources is often enough to answer a question about the evidence for clinical practice. If it still proves necessary to locate primary studies, there are systems in place in PubMed to help retrieve high-quality articles. It is not possible to go into precise detail within the limits of this chapter, but Bidwell (2004) provides a comprehensive guide to searching PubMed, using features such as the 'clinical queries' mode, which can assist in reducing the volume of information often obtained when performing a simple search. PubMed also provides excellent online tutorials. For those wanting to expand their skills in evidence-based practice, CASP provides a wide variety of educational tools and resources. ScHARR is also worth a visit. It provides an introduction to evidence-based practice on the internet, 'Netting the Evidence', with links to helpful organisations and useful learning resources. All the above resources should help to make searches more fruitful and less frustrating.

KEY POINTS

- A number of steps are involved in applying an evidence-based approach to practice.
- Database searching can be difficult without having specific training.
- Accessing secondary (evaluated) sources of evidence such as evidence-based guidelines and systematic reviews can often answer your question quickly and effectively.
- Evidence-based guidelines generally provide condition-specific advice and clear guidance for practitioners.

FURTHER AREAS TO CONSIDER

- How do you ensure that you keep your practice up to date and in line with the latest evidence?
- Access some of the websites provided in this chapter and compare the evidence to your current practice.
- Remember to take into account individual patient/client issues when applying evidence: is it the most suitable method for that person?
- Always discuss the evidence with your individual patients, including possible side effects, and provide them with the necessary information to enable them to make an informed decision.

CHAPTER 9

CASE SCENARIOS

OVERVIEW

This chapter provides both straightforward and more complex case scenarios for the reader to work through, relating to some of the long-term conditions (LTCs) seen in primary care. **Part One** considers care management issues for people with a specific LTC. **Part Two** considers care management issues for those with more complex needs. As in earlier chapters, pauses for reflection are provided for each scenario. A suggested course of action is then supplied for each scenario. In practice each person's individual health and cultural and social needs should be taken into consideration when planning care.

INTRODUCTION

The aim of this chapter is to draw together some of the issues that have now been discussed throughout this book and put them into practice through a case study approach. Case scenarios will be provided relating to various conditions, beginning with straightforward cases and progressing to more complex issues. Although based on actual patients, all names and identifying details have been anonymised to ensure confidentiality. You are encouraged to read through these and develop an appropriate care plan; based on the information you have read so far and through accessing the relevant evidence-based guideline for the condition being discussed. This may be done as an individual or group learning exercise. Following each scenario, suggested courses of action are provided which are based on appropriate evidence-based guidelines. Remember that in practice each person you see will have individual physical, cultural and social needs; it is impossible to cover all potential scenarios, so the ones provided are meant as a guide to assist you in putting theory into practice. Assessment of each person through taking a comprehensive history and carrying out a physical examination (where indicated) will ensure that you determine individual need. This should then be built into a care management plan agreed by both yourself and the person with the LTC, that should incorporate education and advice on self-management.

PART ONE: CASE SCENARIOS

Respiratory: asthma

The suggested answers to the asthma scenarios are based on information taken from the latest edition of the British Thoracic Society (BTS)/SIGN (2008) *British Guideline on the Management of Asthma*. For further in-depth information you should access the full version of the guideline or the guideline currently appropriate for your country.

Scenario 1

Bob is a 33-year-old male teacher, who recently had an asthma exacerbation while socialising with friends after work. He presented at the A&E (accident and emergency) department of his local general hospital, where he was admitted and transferred to the acute medical admissions unit. On admission Bob found it difficult to complete sentences and his peak expiratory flow (PEF) was 40 per cent of that predicted (no record was available to hospital staff of his best PEF). His respiratory rate was 27/minute and his heart rate 115/minute. Transfer to the intensive care unit (ICU) for ventilation was discussed, but after instigation of an appropriate treatment plan, his condition stabilised and ventilation was not necessary. He was transferred to a medical ward, from which he was discharged three days later and advised to attend the asthma clinic run in his general practice for treatment review. When reviewing his notes prior to his appointment, the nurse responsible for asthma care in the practice noted that he had not attended for review for over a year, despite two reminder letters. It was also discovered that he had not been collecting his prescriptions for his steroid preventer inhalers for over a year but had been collecting his short-term acting beta 2 agonist reliever inhalers twice a month.

PAUSE FOR REFLECTION

1   How would you describe Bob's recent asthma exacerbation?
2   What questions do you need to ask him in order to ensure that you take a comprehensive history?
3   Referring to an appropriate evidence-based guideline (e.g. BTS asthma guidelines), develop an appropriate treatment plan for Bob.
4   What general management issues relating to the care of patients with asthma are involved in this scenario?
5   How might you prevent future incidences of this type?

SUGGESTED COURSE OF ACTION

1   Bob's asthma exacerbation can be described as acute severe, although in view of the possibility that ventilation was discussed, the hospital notes should be reviewed to determine whether they were concerned at any time that Bob's exacerbation was life-threatening. The presence of features such as exhaustion, confusion, feeble respiratory effort, or reduced oxygen saturation (SpO2) levels < 92 per cent would have indicated a life-threatening attack. People with a history of a life-threatening attack are known to be at increased risk of mortality.

2   A clear and comprehensive history should be obtained from Bob that should include ascertaining:

   • whether there have been any changes in Bob's work or home life that have caused his asthma to worsen;
   • why he stopped taking his preventer inhalers;
   • whether he understands the difference between his preventer and reliever inhalers;
   • whether he smokes, or is subject to a smoky atmosphere at home;
   • whether there was any particular reason why he stopped attending asthma review;
   • whether his asthma has prevented him from taking part in his usual activities.

3   Bob's inhaler technique should be reviewed and his PEF rate measured. His best or predicted PEF should be clearly noted. The difference between preventer and reliever therapy should be discussed so that Bob

continued

is aware of the difference. Any concerns Bob has regarding the use of preventer therapy (either financial or concern about the effect of steroids) should be clearly addressed. If any lifestyle changes are identified these should also be discussed along with ways of alleviating or minimising the effects of these changes. If Bob is smoking, smoking cessation advice should be given. Bob should be encouraged to self-monitor, provided with a peak flow meter and diary and advised what he should do if his PEF measurements reduce. Bob should be advised that effective asthma control means having no day- or night-time symptoms, no exacerbations, no need for rescue medications and no limitations on normal activity with minimal side effects. If Bob finds it difficult to attend the asthma clinic, alternative arrangements should be discussed. A written self-management plan should be developed that suits Bob's needs, including appropriate review times. As Bob has not been taking his normal preventer inhalers he will need to restart these and then be reviewed at appropriate time intervals to ensure that good control has been achieved and maintained.

4   Despite ordering excessive amounts of reliever therapy and stopping his medication therapy Bob was not reviewed in time to prevent a severe asthma exacerbation. Although Bob had two recall letters no further action was taken. The practice protocol should be reviewed to determine what systems are in place to identify and review people with asthma who are using excessive amounts of reliever therapy or who have stopped their preventer medication suddenly. The team should discuss what would be the best course of action to prevent this scenario from happening again and what systems could be instigated to contact people who do not attend for review despite recall letters. In this particular scenario, in view of the amount of reliever medication Bob had been using, along with the fact that he had stopped taking his preventer medication, an alert should have been generated to ensure that he was either contacted by telephone to come in for review or even visited at home.

Scenario 2

Mary is a 35-year-old woman who has had asthma since the age of 17. She is normally well controlled with 200mg of inhaled steroid used twice daily. She attends clinic for a regular six-monthly review and keeps a peak flow diary. She rarely uses her short-term acting beta 2 agonist reliever inhaler, but recently has begun to do so more often and her peak flow readings have become more variable. She has recently started to walk to work, following a house move, to improve her fitness levels and has noticed increased shortness of breath during her walk. However, after a recent week's holiday she felt much better.

Mary has been called for an early review following an alert system where the nurse running the asthma clinic is alerted to more frequent requests for reliever medication.

PAUSE FOR REFLECTION

1 How would you describe Mary's recent asthma exacerbation?
2 What type of questions would you ask Mary at the review?
3 What else should the review include?
4 If there is nothing obvious in the history that has caused Mary's symptom deterioration what would be the next step?

SUGGESTED COURSE OF ACTION

1 A clear and comprehensive history needs to be taken to determine if there are any underlying reasons for Mary's symptom exacerbation. This should ascertain whether she has changed her job, or whether anything at work has changed that might have affected her control. The fact that her control improved when on holiday could be an indication that either something at work or something at home is exacerbating her condition. As she has recently moved house it is worth enquiring whether she has acquired any pets or whether the previous owner had pets. If Mary has suffered from pet allergies in the past and the previous owner had pets, she may need to consider replacing any carpets or soft furnishings left by the previous owner. If you suspect that a change in the work environment is the cause, Mary should be referred to a chest or occupational physician and serial PEF measurements should be performed at least four times daily. Occupations that are considered high risk include: baking, pastry making, spray painting, animal laboratory work, health care and dental care, food processing, welding, soldering, metalwork, wood-work, chemical processing, textile, plastics and rubber manufacturing, and farming and other jobs with exposure to dusts and fumes (BTS/SIGN 2008).
2 The review should also include checking Mary's inhaler technique, reviewing her PEF and comparing that to her predicted or best and

continued

reviewing her PEF diary to ascertain if there is any pattern to the variability. Ask Mary if there is any possibility she may be pregnant, as pregnancy can also affect asthma control.

3   If there is nothing from the history that appears to have caused Mary's symptom exacerbation then it is likely that the exercise-induced symptoms are a general indication of poorly controlled asthma. Her regular treatment should be reviewed and the next step, step 3 BTS guidelines, would be the addition of a long-term acting beta 2 agonist (LABA). If Mary's symptoms improve with the LABA, this can be continued; if there is some improvement but control is still inadequate then the LABA should be continued and her steroid inhaler dose increased. If there is no improvement the LABA should be stopped and her inhaled steroid increased. If control remains poor, an alternative add-on treatment such as a leukotriene receptor antagonist or modified release theophylline should be considered before moving to step 4 BTS guidelines, namely increasing inhaled corticosteroids to maximum dose. If Mary's PEF diary indicates that it is just the exercise that exacerbates her symptoms and she is otherwise well controlled, the use of an inhaled short-term acting beta 2 agonist before exercise may relieve her symptoms.

Respiratory: chronic obstructive pulmonary disease (COPD)

The suggested answer to the COPD scenario is based on information taken from the NICE (2004d) guideline *Management of Chronic Obstructive Pulmonary Disease in Adults in Primary and Secondary Care*. These were due for an update at the time of publication. For further in-depth information you should access the latest full version of the guideline, or the guideline currently appropriate for your country.

Scenario 3

Karen is a 53-year-old woman who has smoked since the age of 17. She currently smokes 20 cigarettes a day. She has recently developed a chronic productive cough which is particularly bad in the mornings and she has become breathless when climbing stairs. A recent chest x-ray showed no abnormalities. She has been prescribed a short-term acting bronchodilator inhaler to use when needed and advised to attend the respiratory clinic.

PAUSE FOR REFLECTION

1   What diagnosis should be considered for Karen?
2   When taking a comprehensive history, what specific symptoms should you ask Karen about?
3   What tests should be carried out to ascertain a diagnosis?
4   Once diagnosis has been established, what initial advice should be given and what treatment should be considered?

SUGGESTED COURSE OF ACTION

1   In people over the age of 35 who present with any of these symptoms – exertional breathlessness; chronic cough; regular sputum production; frequent winter 'bronchitis'; wheeze; and who have a risk factor (generally smoking) – a diagnosis of COPD should be considered. Karen should also be asked if she has any of the following symptoms: weight loss; effort intolerance; waking at night; ankle swelling; fatigue; occupational hazards; chest pain; haemoptysis. Breathlessness should be graded according to exertion. An up-to-date smoking history should be documented.

2   Spirometry should be performed to ascertain diagnosis and degree of airflow obstruction. Karen has had a chest x-ray; she should also have a full blood count to identify anaemia or polycythaemia and a body mass index (BMI) calculated. If the BMI is < 20 or > 25, dietetic referral should be made. Other tests may be necessary, dependent on symptoms (e.g. sputum culture if sputum is persistently present and purulent). If there has been a significant improvement with the bronchodilator, inhaler > 400ml response, a diagnosis of asthma will need to be excluded.

3   Smoking cessation should discussed with Karen and appropriate support offered, including nicotine replacement therapy. The effect of the short acting bronchodilator that Karen had been prescribed should be assessed by asking whether there has been any improvement in symptoms, activities of daily living, exercise capacity and rapidity of symptom relief. Annual influenza and a (once-only) pneumococcal vaccination should be offered and a self-management plan instigated. The self-management plan should contain advice on how to recognise early signs of an exacerbation and medication and lifestyle issues to prevent exacerbations. Karen should be advised that she should be assessed before any planned air travel. Appropriate review should be arranged.

PAUSE FOR REFLECTION

At Karen's next review she is still symptomatic. Two months after beginning her therapy trial she is still coughing and experiencing some breathlessness. What would be the next course of treatment?

SUGGESTED COURSE OF ACTION

If Karen remains breathless and/or has exercise limitation, consider combining the short-acting bronchodilator agents (beta 2 agonist and anti-muscarinic), or adding in a long-acting bronchodilator (long-acting beta 2 agonist or a long-acting anti-muscarinic). If the cough and sputum production are causing more problems a mucolytic can be added and continued if there is improvement. If still symptomatic, a combination of a long acting beta agonist and inhaled corticosteroid can be offered but should be discontinued if there is no benefit within four weeks. Once Karen's symptoms are stabilised she should be reviewed at least annually. This should comprise a review of smoking status and medication; including concordance and inhaler technique, BMI, symptom review, and determination of any signs of complications such as respiratory failure and depression. Spirometry should be reviewed annually. Pulmonary rehabilitation should be considered in all people who consider themselves functionally disabled.

Diabetes

The suggested answers to the diabetes scenarios are based on information taken from the NICE (2008) guideline *Diabetes – Type 2*. For further in-depth information you should access the latest full version of the guideline, or the guideline currently appropriate for your country.

Scenario 4

Jennifer is a 49-year-old woman who was diagnosed with type 2 diabetes two years ago. Jennifer lives with her 25-year-old daughter who has learning disabilities and also cares for her elderly mother. Jennifer struggles with her weight and her BMI is currently 29. Jennifer was started on the biguanide Metformin one year ago and her dose has since been increased to 500mg three times daily. She is also taking 75mg aspirin once daily, an ACE (angiotensin-converting enzyme) inhibitor once daily for her blood pressure and a daily statin for her cholesterol. Jennifer does not monitor her blood sugars as she finds it stressful to do and upsetting when her readings are raised. Jennifer is attending for her annual review; her blood results, taken prior to the appointment, indicate that her HbA1c is raised at 8 per cent and her total cholesterol is 5.5. All other results are within normal limits. Jennifer's blood pressure is raised at 145/90. When discussing her diabetes control Jennifer admits that she frequently forgets her tablets and finds it difficult to stick to a healthy eating regime, often resorting to high-calorie, high-fat snacks or fast food. She has little time for exercise due to the time spent caring for her daughter and mother. She has, however, stopped taking sugar in her tea. The GP who reviewed her results prior to the review has suggested an increase in both her oral hypoglycaemic and cholesterol medication.

PAUSE FOR REFLECTION

1   How can you help Jennifer to improve her diet, lifestyle and con-cordance with medication?
2   Is increasing her medication a sensible thing to do?
3   What other members of the multi-disciplinary team may be able to help?

SUGGESTED COURSE OF ACTION

1   In order to help Jennifer achieve changes in her diet and lifestyle you need to consider what she wants and how you can empower her to make changes (see Chapter 5). Emphasising the positives (i.e. congratulating her on stopping taking sugar in her tea) will help encourage her. Exploring what areas she feels she may be able to change will encourage Jennifer's motivation. For example, although Jennifer finds it difficult to make time to cook, perhaps suggesting she takes her daughter with her when visiting her mother and cooking one healthy meal for all of them may help, rather than cooking for her mother and resorting to fast food for herself. There may be activities that she can do with her daughter that would be beneficial for both of them in increasing her exercise and losing weight. The key is helping

continued

her to explore ways in which she feels she can make changes. Discuss the reasons why she doesn't take her medication: does she not like taking tablets or does she forget? A dosset or pill box may help; a dossett box is used for storing prescribed medicine and tablets. It is normally a hard plastic grid with sliding clear plastic windows that are labelled with days of the week. A dosset box enables the user to take tablets at regular intervals. Perhaps a laminated chart on the wall or fridge in her kitchen may act as a useful reminder.

2   In this scenario, as Jennifer readily admits to forgetting her medication, increasing it is not a sensible choice. How and when people take their medication and how they feel about it should always be discussed before making any changes. What is crucial is to emphasise to Jennifer the importance of taking the correct dosages, ascertain what suits her, and develop a plan that suits her lifestyle and individual need.

3   Jennifer would probably benefit from a review with a dietician who will be able to suggest easy ways in which she can alter her diet to suit her lifestyle (see Chapter 10). Jennifer may also benefit from a referral to social services to see if they can help with caring for her mother and daughter. The local pharmacist may be able to assist with organising an easier method to help Jennifer remember her medication. Assistive technology such as text reminders may be a possibility.

This case scenario demonstrates the importance of developing concordance and understanding people's individual needs rather than simply relying on increasing their medication.

Scenario 5

Jeff is a 36-year-old married man recently diagnosed with type 2 diabetes. He is not taking any medication at present, but was seen by the dietician within a month of diagnosis. Jeff is a long-distance lorry driver and has a young family. He has attended for his first three-monthly review, his HbA1c is 9 per cent (at diagnosis it was 9.1 per cent) and his cholesterol is unchanged at 6.5. His BP remains raised at 150/95 and his BMI is 30. Jeff has a strong family history of both diabetes and cardiovascular disease; his father had diabetes and died of a myocardial infarction at age 59 and his 62-year-old mother, who also has diabetes, has poor eyesight and has had two toes amputated. Jeff readily admits that his diet is poor and that when he is not driving he drinks between eight and ten pints of beer in the evenings. He feels that developing diabetes was inevitable and that there is little he can do about it.

PAUSE FOR REFLECTION

1   What sort of advice and support can you give Jeff?
2   What pharmacological treatment, if any, would you advise for Jeff?
3   When would be a suitable time for the next review?

SUGGESTED COURSE OF ACTION

1   Jeff is clearly having difficulties coming to terms with the diagnosis and is influenced by his experience of the condition so far. Jeff would benefit from referral to a structured programme of diabetes education that his wife could attend as well. This could be through a locally run scheme such as DESMOND (Diabetes Education and Self Management for Ongoing and Newly Diagnosed Diabetes) if available, or referral to an Expert Patient Programme. If a suitable programme is not available in your area it is important to develop a structured education programme for Jeff, to ensure that he is fully aware of his condition and potential complications, and how these can be avoided with appropriate lifestyle changes. The aim should be not only to improve his knowledge and skills but also to motivate him to effectively self-manage. As with Jennifer, you need to empower and support Jeff to make changes to his diet and lifestyle through exploring how he feels about the diagnosis and what changes he feels he could make. Inviting Jeff to bring his wife to the consultation may also be helpful, as he may have found it difficult to discuss with her the diagnosis and the potential implications of having diabetes. Jeff will need particular support in assisting him in making dietary changes and reducing his alcohol intake on his rest days. Jeff should be asked about any potential problems with his diabetes, such as erectile dysfunction, neuropathy and/or depression, so that these can be dealt with appropriately.
2   In view of Jeff's weight, metformin would be suitable first line therapy in achieving normoglycaemia, providing his renal function tests are normal. Although Jeff has not altered his lifestyle at this stage it is important to begin the process of glycaemic control. It is imperative that Jeff realises that the medication is to assist him in achieving normo-glycaemia and is not a 'quick fix'. Jeff also needs to be prescribed an ACE inhibitor for his blood pressure (BP) which has been consistently raised, and a statin for his cholesterol, as his cardiovascular risk profile

continued

is poor. Jeff should be offered low-dose aspirin 75mg daily as he has significant cardiovascular risk factors (family history, hypertension, features of the metabolic syndrome). How and when to take his medication should be incorporated into a personalised treatment plan.

3   Jeff needs to be seen in a month to assess his BP. A lipid profile and HbA1c should be repeated in three months, followed by a review. Jeff should also be supported in the interim to encourage him in making lifestyle changes and this will depend on his individual need.

Musculoskeletal: osteoporosis

The suggested answer to the osteoporosis scenario is based on information taken from the CKS (2006c) clinical topic *Osteoporosis*. For further in-depth information you should access the latest evidence-based summary or the guideline currently appropriate for your country.

Scenario 6

Mrs T is an active 79-year-old woman who has attended for review at her GP surgery, following recent hospitalisation and rehabilitation for a fragility hip fracture, which occurred when she had a simple fall at home after getting out of bed. Apart from the fracture, Mrs T, who lives on her own, has little other medical history of note; however, her BMI is low at 19. Prior to the fracture she was extremely independent. At the time of consultation she is staying with her daughter but is keen to return home as soon as she is able.

PAUSE FOR REFLECTION

1   What condition may have caused Mrs T's fracture?
2   What other tests may you need to carry out to confirm your diagnosis?
3   What treatment and advice should be offered to Mrs T?

SUGGESTED COURSE OF ACTION

1   Although in general a diagnosis of osteoporosis is made by measuring bone mineral density (BMD), in Mrs T's case she has had a fragility fracture from a standing height and is over age 75, so a diagnosis of osteoporosis can be assumed.

2   There is no need for BMD measurement. However, differential diagnosis such as skeletal metastases or multiple myeloma should be ruled out, if indicated from the clinical history. If a secondary cause is suspected this should be investigated: for example, thyroid function test to exclude hyperthyroidism, and bone, liver and renal biochemistry to exclude osteomalacia.

3   Mrs T should be started on a biphosphonate and given clear verbal and written instructions on how to take it. If she has a history of any upper gastrointestinal disorder alendronate should not be used. Dietary intake should be discussed and calcium and vitamin D prescribed if dietary intake is inadequate. Mrs T may also benefit from referral to a dietician to ensure adequate nutritional intake, as she is underweight. She should also be asked if she has had any other falls in the past year and, if so, the frequency, context and characteristics of the falls. A multi-factorial falls risk assessment should be offered if she has had recurrent falls or demonstrates abnormalities of gait or balance. Other lifestyle measures that can help reduce bone thinning should be discussed. These include:

- regular low-impact weight-bearing exercise, such as brisk walking, jogging or dancing;
- smoking cessation (if Mrs T smokes);
- cutting down the amount of alcohol if Mrs T drinks excessively.

Mrs T's daughter should be involved in the consultation to determine whether any extra help is required in enabling Mrs T to return to her home environment as soon as possible. This may involve an occupational therapy assessment or social services support and these should be arranged if deemed necessary.

Musculoskeletal: osteoarthritis

The suggested answer to the osteoarthritis scenario is based on information taken from the CKS (2008b) clinical topic *Osteoarthritis* and the National Collaborating Centre for Chronic Conditions (2008) clinical guideline *Osteoarthritis*. For further in-depth information you should access the latest evidence-based summary or the guideline currently appropriate for your country.

Scenario 7

Mrs Smith, a 69-year-old woman, attends for a review of her osteoarthritis, with which she was diagnosed one year previously. During this time she has developed increasing stiffness and pain in her joints. Pain is a particular problem when walking, and as she also finds it difficult to get in and out of the car she has found herself more and more confined to the house, relying on family and friends to shop for her. She is reluctant to mobilise due to the pain but dislikes taking tablets, so often does not take the painkillers that have been prescribed for her.

PAUSE FOR REFLECTION

1   How would you assess Mrs Smith and what advice can you give her to help improve her quality of life?
2   What analgesia would you suggest?

SUGGESTED COURSE OF ACTION

1   Mrs Smith should be advised that there are options to reduce her pain and disability and she should not suffer silently. Following a full assessment of the severity of the pain and the effect on her quality of life, state of mind, relationships and leisure activities a management plan should be devised that takes into account both her individual needs and any co-morbidities. She should be given verbal and written advice about self-care and treatment options, provided with information about organisations such as Arthritis Care, and referred to a local Expert Patient Programme if available. The importance of a healthy diet should be discussed with Mrs Smith, including referral to a dietician for a nutritional management plan if she is under- or overweight. The importance of regular exercise should be stressed and it should be explained that pain and stiffness will become worse with inactivity. A number of physical treatment options may be considered including referral to a physiotherapist who can advise on strengthening exercises, improvement of aerobic fitness or manual hip therapy such as manipulation and stretching. An occupational therapist or a Disability Equipment Assessment Centre can advise on assistive devices, appropriate footwear, supports and braces, and electrotherapy such as TENS (transcutaneous electrical nerve stimulation).

2   The importance of taking regular analgesia should be stressed to prevent the pain from becoming unbearable, and Mrs Smith should be advised that paracetamol should be taken regularly, not just 'as required'. Topical non-steroidal anti-inflammatory drugs (NSAIDS) can supplement or substitute the paracetamol for knee or hand osteoarthritis. If these methods prove ineffective other options such as oral NSAIDS (to replace the topical NSAID), codeine or topical capsaicin may be considered but the risks and benefits should be considered in individual patients, taking into account factors such as age and co-morbidities; for example, oral NSAIDS should be avoided in patients taking low dose aspirin. Where oral NSAIDS are prescribed they should be used at the lowest effective dose for the shortest possible period of time. Mrs Smith should be reviewed periodically to ensure that treatment is effective.

Skin conditions: eczema

The suggested answer to the following scenario is based on information taken from the CKS (2008a) clinical topic *Eczema*. For further in-depth information you should access the latest evidence-based summary or the guideline currently appropriate for your country.

Scenario 8

Amy, a 20-year-old female student, has attended for an appointment following a recent flare-up of her eczema, which she has had since childhood. Amy has a number of areas of dry skin and redness and has suffered increased itching, which wakes her at night. When reviewing Amy's prescription history you notice that although she has recently been requesting frequent repeat prescriptions for topical corticosteroids she does not appear to have requested regular emollients for some time.

PAUSE FOR REFLECTION

1   What type of things may have triggered Amy's recent flare-up and how would you rule these out?
2   What advice would you give Amy and what treatment would you suggest?

SUGGESTED COURSE OF ACTION

1   The possibility of underlying infection should first be ruled out; this includes eczema herpeticum, viral infections such as varicella (chicken pox) and bacterial infections. Signs and symptoms of eczema herpeticum include possible fever and lethargy, areas of rapidly worsening painful eczema, clustered blisters similar to cold sores and punched out erosions; if this is suspected it requires urgent hospital admission. If the eczema is weeping and crusted, or if there are signs of pustules, bacterial infection should be diagnosed and an appropriate antibiotic prescribed. Swabbing lesions is unnecessary unless there is a failure to respond to antibiotic treatment. Trigger factors can include stress, change of diet, pets or irritants. As Amy is a student she may have become stressed about exams or perhaps a recent move away from home. A change of detergent or soap may have triggered the flare-up; it is important to determine possible causes through careful history taking so that these can be eliminated.

2   Amy should be advised about the avoidance of possible trigger factors and asked to consider what may have caused the exacerbation. While experiencing the flare-up a moderate potency topical corticosteroid, either cream or ointment depending on Amy's preference, should be used on inflamed areas for 48 hours after signs and symptoms have resolved. Emollients should be used frequently and liberally, and the importance of regular use should be discussed with Amy, rather than relying on topical corticosteroids during a flare-up. Sedating antihistamines can be prescribed if itching is affecting sleep but ensure Amy is not in the middle of exams. Amy should be advised that once the current flare-up is under control topical corticosteroid treatment should be stepped down. Options include: using the lowest potency and amount of topical corticosteroid necessary to maintain control, using topical corticosteroids on two consecutive days once a week (weekend therapy) on any specific patches of skin that frequently flare up, or a one-month trial on non-sedating antihistamines if Amy is suffering severe itching or urticaria (although there is limited evidence for this approach). Emollients should be used frequently and liberally at all times, even when the skin is clear. The importance of not scratching and keeping fingernails short to avoid scratching while asleep should be emphasised. Amy should be seen once the current exacerbation is under control to review treatment.

PART TWO: COMPLEX CASE SCENARIOS

People with more complex needs

Scenario 9

Mr Evans is a 78-year-old ex-miner who suffers from advanced COPD and cardiovascular disease (CVD). He is on home oxygen therapy and uses a nebuliser. He has had three admissions to hospital in the past year for exacerbation of his COPD.

PAUSE FOR REFLECTION

1 What sort of management would be most suitable for Mr Evans?
2 What members of the nursing team would be best suited to provide care for Mr Evans?

SUGGESTED COURSE OF ACTION

1 In view of the number of admissions and type of treatment Mr Evans is receiving, he would be classed as end stage COPD and an appropriate package of care should be organised. This may be through referral to a hospital at home scheme, the district nursing team or through a case management approach if this is available in your area. Mr Evans' needs are complex and at this stage a discussion about palliative care services should be broached. As the disease advances a clear management plan based on Mr Evans' and his carer's wishes should be implemented; this may be in the form of a care management pathway for people at the end of life.

2 Mr Evans' care needs would be best met by either the district nursing service, who have the appropriate training and experience and are well placed to manage and support people requiring palliative care, or a community matron with experience of end-of-life care. Respiratory specialist nurses can provide invaluable support and advice regarding maximising symptom control. Palliative care specialist nurses may also be involved in the care package.

Scenario 10

Mrs Jones is a 92-year-old woman who has osteoarthritis, COPD, cardiovascular disease and heart failure. She lives alone, and until recently had been relatively independent. Within the past year she has had a number of falls, which have resulted in numerous hospital admissions. It has been suggested that she moves into a residential care home. Mrs Jones is keen to return to her own home but has agreed that she needs extra support.

PAUSE FOR REFLECTION

1   What type of care would be the most suitable for Mrs Jones?
2   What types of skills would the nurse responsible for Mrs Jones' care require?
3   How can the nurse responsible for her care help maximise the quality of Mrs Jones' care?

SUGGESTED COURSE OF ACTION

1   Mrs Jones has complex care needs and is at high risk of repeated admission to hospital. She has a number of co-morbidities and will consequently be taking a number of different medications. Enabling her to remain at home requires a case management approach to her care to coordinate a health and social care package that meets her specific needs. The principles behind case management include enabling Mrs Jones to have a personalised care plan based on her individual needs and choice, and to ensure that appropriate referral is made to the correct agencies and health and social care professionals when it is needed.
2   In order to provide the care that Mrs Jones requires, the nurse responsible for her case management will need a number of key skills, including:

    •   advanced level assessment skills;
    •   supplementary or independent prescribing qualification;
    •   health promotion skills;
    •   the ability to coordinate care across agencies;
    •   the ability to support self-care and independence;
    •   leadership and management skills.

Once Mrs Jones has been assessed and a care plan developed, the nurse responsible for Mrs Jones' case management will need to:

- work in partnership with Mrs Jones' GP and other agencies, such as social services;
- work collaboratively with other professionals, carers and relatives;
- make regular contact with Mrs Jones;
- order investigations where necessary;
- update medical records;
- ensure Mrs Jones is prescribed and receives appropriate medication;
- educate Mrs Jones, her carers and relatives about her condition and how to identify exacerbations;
- liaise with secondary care;
- prepare Mrs Jones and her family for any condition changes and support choices about end-of-life care when this proves necessary.

Scenario 11

Tim is 35 years old. He has epilepsy and learning disabilities and was diagnosed with type 2 diabetes three years ago for which he remains diet controlled. He lives with his mother and his sister (his main carer) and attends a centre on a daily basis where he enjoys carpentry and is relatively independent. However, he has had one hospital admission in the past year, following hitting his head at the centre after suffering a seizure. His sister is concerned that Tim's weight is creeping up, despite eating healthily at home. His BMI has gone up from 27 to 29 within the past two years. Tim is attending the surgery for an annual review of both his epilepsy and diabetes.

PAUSE FOR REFLECTION

1   What type of care would be most suitable for Tim?
2   What types of issues need to be discussed in Tim's review?
3   What other nurses and health care professionals may be helpful in providing advice to Tim and his family?

SUGGESTED COURSE OF ACTION

1   Tim would be best managed through a disease/care management approach for high-risk patients, with a multidisciplinary team providing high-quality evidence-based care to achieve optimum health and reduce risks of complications and deterioration. The nurse conducting Tim's review should ensure that the information from the review is shared between the necessary health care professionals involved in Tim's care, Tim and his carer.

2   Tim's review will need to consider issues related to both his epilepsy and diabetes, including prior measurement of all physical parameters relating to the diabetes review. Regarding his epilepsy Tim and his sister should be asked about seizure control, adverse effects of medication and compliance with medication. As Tim has been admitted during the past year following a seizure it should be ensured that he is taking his medication correctly, whether he was reviewed by an epilepsy specialist following his admission and what his control has been like since. If Tim's epilepsy appears to be inadequately controlled specialist advice should be sought; an epilepsy specialist nurse is a useful resource. Regular blood test monitoring is not recommended in epilepsy unless specifically indicated (CKS 2006b). Tim and his sister should be provided with a general care plan that includes advice re lifestyle issues relating to both his epilepsy and diabetes. Regarding the diabetes, a full annual review should be carried out. This should include a full medical examination including a review of all his blood tests to determine any possible complications, BP, foot screening, a check to see whether he has had his annual retinal screening and medication review. Tim and his carer's understanding of diabetes should be assessed and support given.

3   In view of Tim's recent weight gain a referral to a dietician who can help in the development of a personal nutrition plan is recommended. Tim and his carer can then discuss this with the day centre that Tim attends to ensure consistency. Tim and his carer should be provided with the contact details of an epilepsy specialist nurse who can advise about seizure control and any other measures that need to be taken to maintain Tim's safety. Tim would also benefit from referral to a community learning disabilities nurse who could liaise between him and his family, the day centre and the surgery to ensure that he is receiving the same advice and care from all sources.

CONCLUSION

Having now completed the case scenarios in this chapter you should have a better understanding of the type of care management that is suitable for individual people with LTCs. These include people who can become active participants in their own care, high-risk patients who need extra support to maximise health outcomes and highly complex patients with co-morbidities and complex conditions who would benefit from a case management approach to care. You should also be able to translate information from evidence-based guidelines and care pathways into realistic goals and care packages for individual patients. Remember to continually update your practice as new research becomes available and ensure that the evidence you use is up to date and relevant for your client group. The importance of a multi-disciplinary approach to care cannot be over-emphasised, likewise the importance of sharing information to avoid duplication or omission of care. Although the case studies are purposefully generic and have not covered any particular cultural or social issues, you should consider the specific needs in your area and incorporate these into your care planning and implementation.

KEY POINTS

- Assess each patient on an individual basis and take into account cultural and social as well as health needs.
- Ensure that you have a method within your practice area to identify people requiring a disease/care management or case management approach.
- Incorporate advice on self-management into individual care plans.

FURTHER AREAS TO CONSIDER

- Where case management schemes are not available, who takes responsibility for people with complex care needs?
- How do you ensure that records are shared between appropriate health and social care professionals?
- If you are providing a disease/care management or case management approach, how do you ensure that your educational needs are met?

CHAPTER 10

NUTRITIONAL AND MEDICATION MANAGEMENT

OVERVIEW

The importance of multi-disciplinary teamworking was discussed in Chapter 3. This chapter will explore the importance of dietary and medicines management in the care of people with a long-term condition (LTC).

Part One: Nutritional management. The relationship between obesity and LTCs is explored and practical guidelines provided relating to assessment and management of a patient's nutritional status, including why weight management advice is important.

Part Two: Medication management. Department of Health (DoH) figures indicate that 50 per cent of patients with LTCs fail to take their medicines properly. Schemes that have been shown to be successful in encouraging patients to take their medicines correctly are reviewed, along with the importance of teamworking with pharmacists.

INTRODUCTION

This book has so far explored the ways in which nurses working in the primary care environment can support people with LTCs. The importance of team-working and appropriate referral has also been discussed as well as the need for a coordinated and systematic approach to care. The aim of this chapter is to discuss two particularly important aspects of LTC care: nutrition and medicines management. Part One of this chapter, written by a qualified dietician, reviews the relationship between obesity and LTCs, focusing on aetiology, associated health risks and management. Part Two reviews the importance of medicines management and the importance of the role of the pharmacist in educating and supporting people with LTCs.

PART ONE: NUTRITIONAL MANAGEMENT OF PATIENTS WITH LTCS

Poor nutrition can be both the cause and a cause of concern in many patients suffering from an LTC. Successful dietary intervention can reduce the risk of further complications and improve quality of life. All health care professionals working in primary care should be able to identify patients in need of dietary evaluation and have an obligation to include other members of the multi-disciplinary team within each individual care plan, to offer appropriate advice and support. A dietician should be involved with the care of these patients in order to assist them to address and achieve their nutritional needs.

Obesity and long-term conditions

The incidence of obesity, in the UK and worldwide, is increasing rapidly with no sign of slowing down. In 2005 the Health Survey for England showed that there has been a dramatic increase in obesity in the UK from 7 per cent in 1980 to 23 per cent in 2003. The Department of Health equates this to approximately 24 million adults in the UK being classed as obese in 2005 (DoH 2005e). In addition, rates of childhood obesity are also rising, with 16 per cent of boys and girls aged 2 to 15 being classed as obese and almost one-third as either overweight or obese (DoH 2005e). It is generally agreed that overweight children tend to become overweight adults; therefore these figures have serious implications for the future health of the nation.

Obesity is classed as one of the biggest causes of mortality and morbidity in the UK (National Obesity Forum 2008). Obesity is also strongly associated with other medical problems, notably the chronic diseases/long-term conditions highlighted in this book (see Table 10.1). It is vital therefore that the patient understands that obesity is a clinical term with health implications rather than just a question of how someone looks (NICE 2006b).

Table 10.1 Health risks of obesity

Greatly increased risk	Moderately increased risk	Slightly increased risk
Type 2 diabetes	Cardiovascular diseases	Certain cancers; including colon, kidney, prostate (men), post-menopausal breast and endometrial (women)
Gallbladder disease	Hypertension	Reproductive hormone abnormalities
Dyslipidaemia	Osteoarthritis (knee)	Polycystic Ovary Syndrome
Insulin resistance	Hyperuricaemia and gout	Impaired fertility
Breathlessness		Lower back pain
Sleep apnoea		Increases anaesthetic risk
		Foetal defects associated with maternal obesity

(adapted from Thomas and Bishop 2007)

PAUSE FOR REFLECTION

What impact has obesity had on the incidence of LTCs in your area?

Classification of obesity

Body mass index (BMI) is a widely used and recognised measurement of weight for height in adults. It is defined as weight in kilograms divided by height in metres squared (kg/m^2). From this, worldwide classifications of obesity can be determined (see Table 10.2). However, results should be interpreted as a rough guide, as the BMI does not take into consideration muscle mass and therefore the degree of fatness between individuals. Anthropometric measurements may also be used. More recently, waist circumference has been used as an alternative classification system. A high proportion of abdominal fat is related to an increased health risk, notably of type 2 diabetes and cardiovascular disease (see Table 10.3). NICE obesity guidelines (2006b) state that once measurements are taken, the classification should be told to the patient and the long-term health risks explained.

Table 10.2 Classification of overweight and obesity

Classification	BMI (kg/m^2)
Healthy weight	18.5–24.9
Overweight	25–29.9
Obesity I	30–34.9
Obesity II	35–39.9
Obesity III	40 or more

Table 10.3 Waist circumference and risk factors

	Increased risk	Substantial risk
Men	≥ 94cm (~37 inches)	≥ 102cm (~40 inches)
Women	≥ 80cm (~32 inches)	≥ 88cm (~35 inches)

(adapted from WHO 1998)

Aetiology of obesity

In theory obesity is the simple consequence of an imbalance of energy input to energy output (i.e. a positive energy balance). It is generally considered to be the consequence of energy-rich, nutrient-poor diets and sedentary lifestyles. In reality there are many influencing factors on this equation and all aspects of a patient's diet and lifestyle should be considered in order to make appropriate interventions. Genetic influences on obesity are widely discussed and some research has shown familial characteristics between overweight parents and their children. There are also a small number of single gene disorders such as Prader-Willie syndrome where obesity is noted as a clinical consequence. However, it is evident that obesity is not just the result of a genetic defect but is affected by many factors such as environmental, psychological and social influences. Therefore, with appropriate interventions even subjects with genetic predispositions should be able to maintain their weight within a normal range (Barasi 2003).

PAUSE FOR REFLECTION

What environmental, psychological and social influences impact on the development of obesity?

Management of obesity

Obesity can be managed in primary care by a motivated, well-informed multi-disciplinary team. Recognition and identification of the treatment groups that require further advice and support is the vital first step (see Table 10.4). Initial assessment of the patient using the classifications previously discussed should be the first line of action before moving on to discuss possible interventions with the patient. Other information to collect includes personal medical history, family history, social history, past history of dieting, readiness to change, barriers to change, and current diet and levels of activity (BDA 1997). Guidelines on the first steps of managing obesity may be found in NICE *Guideline 43* (2006b) and the National Obesity Forum (2008).

Table 10.4 Treatment groups

Treatment or advice should be offered to:

- patients with a BMI of 30 or above
- patients with a BMI of 28 and above with co-morbidities (e.g. CHD, diabetes)
- patients with any degree of overweight coinciding with diabetes, other severe risk factors or serious disease
- patients who self-refer where appropriate.

Special consideration should be given to:

- parents of families with more than one overweight or obese member.

Preventive advice should be offered to high-risk individuals:

- patients with a family history of obesity
- smokers
- patients with learning difficulties
- low-income groups.

(adapted from National Obesity Forum 2008)

There are several treatment options for obesity, but all are underpinned with achieving an energy balance with healthy eating advice and promotion of regular exercise. Multi-component interventions should be put in place to encourage sustainable lifestyle changes. Other interventions such as drug treatment and surgery are only to be considered after three to six months if the first line treatments (i.e. diet and lifestyle changes) are not considered successful. Success can be determined by a reduction in BMI or waist circumference and/or improvement of symptoms and reduced markers of co-morbidities. Guidance on who is appropriate for second line interventions is outlined in Table 10.5.

Management of all patients should involve as many members of the primary care team as possible and available. Guidance should be consistent and

Table 10.5 A guide to deciding level of intervention

BMI classification	Waist circumference			Co-morbidities present
	Low	High	Very high	
Overweight				
Obesity I				
Obesity II				
Obesity III				

☐ General advice on healthy weight and lifestyle

▨ Diet and physical activity

▨ Diet and physical activity; consider drugs

■ Diet and physical activity; consider surgery

(adapted from NICE 2006b)

always patient-centred, with the individual patient goals at the centre of all discussions. Members of a team that can be involved include doctors, nurses, dieticians, counsellors, health trainers and physiotherapists. All these team members should familiarise themselves with relevant information from local community services that can be passed to the patient including local leisure facilities for exercise programmes, weight management groups for group support and any healthy food schemes (e.g. fruit and vegetable boxes).

PAUSE FOR REFLECTION

Do you know what schemes are available in your area? If so, how do you ensure you inform your patients/clients?

Targets of treatment

Achievable, realistic weight loss goals should be set with the patient. It is recognised that a 5 to 10 per cent loss of original weight can bring about substantial benefits to health (Table 10.6). A maximum loss of 0.5 to 1kg per week is ideal. This is achieved by maintaining a deficit of 500 to 600kcals per day to ensure sustainable weight loss. This weight loss should be ideally occur within three months and maintained for 12 months as an indicator of success (NICE 2006b).

Table 10.6 Benefits of a 10kg weight loss in a 100kg individual, i.e. 10% weight loss

Indication	Improvement to health
Mortality	> 20% ↓ total mortality > 30% ↓ diabetes-related deaths > 40% ↓ obesity-related cancers
Blood pressure	10 mmHg ↓ systolic 20 mmHg ↓ diastolic
Lipids	10% total cholesterol 15% ↓ low-density lipoprotein 30% ↓ triglycerides 8% ↑ high-density lipoprotein
Diabetes	30–50% ↓ fasting glucose 50% ↓ risk of diabetes developing 15% ↓ in HbA1c
Physical complications	Improved back and joint pain Improved lung function Reduced frequency of sleep apnoea

(adapted from Jung 1997)

KEY RESOURCES

- NICE *Clinical Guideline 43: Obesity* (2006b)
- National Obesity Forum (NOF): www.nationalobesityforum.org.uk
- International Obesity Task Force (2003): www.iotf.org
- British Dietetic Association (BDA) Weight Wise Campaign: www.bda weightwise.com
- Food Standards Agency: www.food.gov.uk
- Department of Health: www.doh.gov.uk

KEY POINTS

- Obesity rates in the UK are increasing for both adults and children.
- Obesity is a serious health risk with strong links to many chronic diseases.
- The level of obesity and associated health risks can be determined by BMI and waist circumference.
- Gradual, realistic weight loss goals should be set with the patient to achieve sustainable lifestyle changes.
- Dietary modification and exercise promotion are the basis of weight management.
- Medications and surgery may be suitable for some patients.
- Ten per cent weight loss can bring about substantial improvements to health.

FURTHER AREAS TO CONSIDER

- What other nutritional needs may people with LTCs present with?
- What, if any, assessment tools do you use to assess people with nutritional needs?

PART TWO: MEDICATION MANAGEMENT

Effective medicines management is a vital cog in the wheel in the effective care of people with LTCs. Use of medicines is the most common therapeutic intervention in the NHS; in England alone it is estimated that 20 per cent of Primary Care Trusts' (PCT) funds are spent on medicines and related services each year. However, medicines are also associated with numerous problems; these include the facts that:

- 5 to 17 per cent of hospital admissions are due to medication problems
- 36 per cent of people over the age of 75 are taking more than four medicines
- Medicines are not always prescribed correctly
- Patients do not always use their medicines in the way the prescriber intended, which can result in otherwise avoidable ill-health and waste
- Up to 50 per cent of people with LTCs (many who are elderly) do not take their medicines as prescribed
- It is estimated that £100 million is wasted in the United Kingdom each year on incorrectly prescribed or used medicines
- Medication errors are estimated to cost the NHS £500 million a year in additional days spent in hospital.

(NPC 2002)

The National Prescribing Centre (NPC) is a health service organisation, formed in April 1996 by the Department of Health whose aim is to 'promote and support high quality, cost-effective prescribing and medicines management across the NHS, to help improve patient care and service delivery'. The NPC defines medicines management as 'a system of processes and behaviours that determines how medicines are used, by patients and by the NHS' (NPC 2002). In addition, the NPC notes that medicines management services, which include all aspects of supply and use of medicines, from individual patients to organisations, provide patient-focused care based on need. Examples of medicines management service include:

- Prescription review
- Medication monitoring
- Management of repeat prescribing
- Services to nursing and residential homes
- Patient education.

The *Pharmacy in the Future* document (DoH 2000c) set out a target date of 2004 for the implementation of medicines management schemes in primary care organisations. Since that time a new Community Pharmacy Contractual Framework was put in place in England and Wales in 2005 and a Scottish contract drawn up in 2006 to modernise community pharmacies and to make better use of the skills and knowledge of community pharmacists, enabling them to play a broader role in health care delivery. Some of the schemes that have been put in place by the NPC to meet the original DoH target date and support the implementation of the pharmacy contractual framework in England, Wales and Scotland will be reviewed and summarised below. The overall intention of these schemes was to improve health outcomes, reduce NHS waste and help people get the best from their medicines.

NPC Medicines Management Services (MMS) Collaborative

The overall goal and key aim of the MMS Collaborative is stated on its website (http://www.npc.co.uk/mms/mmsc/index.htm) as follows: 'to help optimise prescribing, plus the experiences and health outcomes for each patient, wherever medicines are involved.'

The MMS stated that it would achieve this aim by:

- Tackling unmet pharmaceutical need
- Helping patients get the best from their medicines, thereby achieving real improvements in health
- Developing innovative and efficient approaches to medicines management services through multi-disciplinary working
- Providing convenient access to medicines management services through multi-disciplinary working which makes better use of pharmacists' skills.

(NPC 2005)

The MMS worked with 146 PCTs throughout England to realise its objectives, which were achieved through a project team, based at the National Prescribing Centre in Liverpool, and local project facilitators appointed by the Primary Care Trust, who utilised a systematic and coordinated programme of quality improvement. The collaborative approach they utilised, developed by the Institute for Healthcare Improvement in the United States, relies on the spread and adoption of existing good practice by people from different backgrounds or organisations working together towards a single, common goal. Four waves of activity took place, beginning with pilot sites participating in a series of learning events, which were combined with local objective setting, action and implementation which took place over a two-year period. Support and consultancy to Wales ended with the conclusion of their last learning workshops and project facilitator sessions, and support and consultancy was provided to one PCT in Scotland. The specific objectives set by the MMS to achieve its aims were:

- Improvements in health through enhanced medicines management, using accepted markers
- A reduction in the waste of medicines
- A reduction in unmet pharmaceutical need in at least one priority area, and an improvement in medicine-taking through the development of patient partnerships
- A reduction in inappropriate clerical and professional time taken up with existing medicines management processes (e.g. in repeat prescribing)
- Improved patient satisfaction with the medicines management services provided.

(NPC 2005)

Local pilot sites were expected to define their own specific measurable targets to achieve these objectives. Some of the key themes that emerged initially from the pilot sites included: prescription review, medication monitoring, improved GP computer and repeat prescribing systems, improved prescription collection and delivery services, and development of concordance between patients and health care professionals.

A collection of monthly measures, through a web-based tool, was used to support the national aims. Measures reviewed included four practice and three organisational measures overall (although some organisational measures had more than one part), full details of which may be obtained from the *MMS Collaborative Wave 3 Review Final Report* (NPC 2005). For example, in phases 2 and 3, one of the practice measures related to determining the percentage of patients aged 65 years or over, regularly taking four or more items of medication, who had had a clinical review of their medication within the past 12 months. An increase in the percentage indicated an improvement. Over a two-year period, the percentage of patients in the target review group who received a documented medication review increased from 29 per cent to 73 per cent (NPC 2005). In phase 4 the percentage of the above reviews where patients were given an explicit opportunity to raise questions and highlight problems about their medicines with an appropriate health care professional was also determined. In addition to the measures the practices were required to submit a self-assessment score in relation to the practice measures indicating whether they were 'getting started' or had achieved 'outstanding sustainable improvement'.

Project facilitators submitted a similar self-assessment score on behalf of their PCT in relation to organisational measures. These included issues such as determining the percentage of patients in registered care homes who had had a documented review of their medicines in the past 12 months in phases 2 and 3. Over a two-year period, the percentage of patients in the target review group who had received a documented medication review increased from 22 per cent to 75 per cent (NPC 2005). The percentage of those documented reviews where the patient was given an explicit opportunity to raise questions and highlight problems about their medicines with an appropriate health care professional was determined in phase 4.

The latest phase of the NPC's approach to improving prescribing, medicines management and the use of medicines in NHS organisations is the Commission for Integrated Medicines Management Programme (CIMM). The aim of this latest programme is to offer the opportunity for primary care commissioners, medicines management and community pharmacy teams, and frontline clinicians to work together with colleagues from around the country on prescribing, medicines management and commissioning issues. The programme will also include the opportunity for participants to focus on the management of a specific LTC.

PAUSE FOR REFLECTION

1 Are there any initiatives going on in your area related to improving medicines management?
2 How do you monitor improvement in your practice?

NPC Community Pharmacy Framework Collaborative (CPFC)

The CPFC was another national initiative supported by the Department of Health and hosted by the MMS team based at the National Prescribing Centre in Liverpool (NPC 2007). Collaborative methodology was used, as previously, to achieve sustainable quality improvement in medicines management for the 28 teams involved (host PCTs in each of the strategic health authorities (SHAs) in England). Project facilitators were recruited by the host PCTs to support the work. The overall goal was stated as follows: 'To realise the benefits of increasing the range and quality of services provided from community pharmacies as an integral part of the NHS.'

Aims included:

- Promoting public health and encouraging self-care through community pharmacies
- To improve health by assessing and attending to the pharmaceutical needs of local people and individual patients
- Increasing patient choice, access and convenience and improving the patient experience
- To develop clinically effective and cost-effective pharmaceutical services that build on the strengths of community pharmacy teams working within a multi-disciplinary environment
- Expanding primary care through commissioning of new medicines management and pharmaceutical services.

(NPC 2007)

The specific objectives set to contribute to these aims included to:

- Increase patient choice
- Increase interventions in long-term conditions
- Reduce medicine-related problems
- Increase public health interventions
- Increase locally commissioned services
- Decrease waste by using interventions
- Decrease the burden on GPs by using interventions.

(NPC 2007)

Programme measures were collected at two levels each month, within individual pharmacies and within the host organisation, to measure improvement activity. There were six pharmacy measures and five spread measures overall (although some measures had more than one part). Full details of all the measures and noteworthy examples from the areas involved may be accessed from the final report (NPC 2007). Examples included pharmacy measure 4: number of face-to-face medicines use reviews (MURs) completed per head of PCT population (increase is an improvement).

The number of MURs, which is part of the advanced level of the community pharmacy contract, increased rapidly and then levelled out. Examples of individual improvements provided in the report included one pharmacy increasing from zero MURs per week to 6.25 MURs per week. Systems put into place by various PCTs to support the pharmacies in achieving these targets included:

- increasing the number of pharmacists accredited to conduct MURs;
- increasing the number of accredited consultation rooms;
- advising community pharmacists to:

  - focus on uncomplicated patients suitable for an MUR;
  - keep the duration of the MUR session to a reasonable time (no more than 15 minutes);
  - increase pharmacists' confidence with tips on interview techniques, body language and taking a positive approach;
  - communicate with GP practices to explain the MUR process and paperwork;
  - explain action GPs should take in response to recommendations on MUR forms;
  - identify the key person and establish a communication process in both the GP practice and pharmacy;
  - highlight the importance for pharmacists to actively get involved with MUR.

Pharmacy measures 4a and 4b were particularly relevant to people with LTCs:

4a The percentage of MURs completed for a long-term condition agreed with the PCT (increase is an improvement).

4b The percentage that reduce medicines waste (increase is an improvement).

As with pharmacy measure 4, MURs increased rapidly and then levelled out. Notable examples included one PCT which used diabetes as its LTC and focused on calibration of glucose meters and people who had more than one meter. Through linking in with Diabetes Week, the PCT launched the service across all local pharmacies, aiding the education programme of encouraging patients to have their meters calibrated annually and raising patients' awareness of the importance of self-care. Pharmacies collected data over a four-week period around patients' current testing, meter usage, meter types and numbers of testing strips being prescribed. The intention was to use these data to provide useful resource material for service development, further patient education programmes and aid in identifying the best way forward to reduce the number of different meters, fluids and glucose strips prescribed.

A number of better practice outcomes related to the CPFC initiative as a whole were noted. In relation to LTCs one PCT which had a high incidence of respiratory disease developed a leaflet to be used as a counselling tool for community pharmacists when dispensing inhalers for patients, particularly those under age 16, with asthma and during MURs. This information could then be taken home by the patient as a resource. The leaflet entitled 'Top Tips for Asthma' was piloted; users liked it but felt stigmatised by the reference to asthma. The leaflet was redeveloped as 'Inhalers . . . Top Tips for Users'. Following further patient evaluation and a 100 per cent positive response from patients who found the leaflet useful and felt that it gave them a better understanding of their inhalers, the leaflet was shared with all community pharmacies and other health care professionals.

This summary has just provided a bird's eye view of the good work and innovative projects that have been developed and supported through the initiative. For further details I strongly recommend you access the full report: *Community Pharmacy Framework Collaborative Final Report* (NPC 2007).

PAUSE FOR REFLECTION

1 What community pharmacy initiatives are you aware of in your area?
2 A key aim of the NPC collaborative programmes is to share good ideas, rather than continually reinventing the wheel; what initiatives could you adopt in your area?

NPC Plus Medicines Partnership Programme

The Medicines Partnership Programme is an initiative aimed at enabling patients to get the most out of their medicines through involving them as partners in decision making about treatment and supporting them in medicine taking. In order to achieve this a process of concordance is used (see also Chapter 4). The NPC describes concordance as 'a process of prescribing and medicine taking based on partnership', although as has been seen earlier in this book concordance has now been expanded to include all aspects of shared decision making between health care professionals and their patients/clients. Compliance measures patient behaviour, the extent to which patients take medicines in accordance with the prescribed instructions, whereas concordance measures a two-way process, involving shared decision making based on partnership which values patients' expertise and beliefs (NPC Plus 2007). In relation to medicine taking, NPC Plus (2007) notes that there are a number of reasons why people do not take their medicines, which include:

- Practical difficulties, such as getting to a pharmacy, opening containers and remembering to take medicines
- Lack of information about their condition and the importance of treatment
- Problems with side effects
- Interference with their daily lives
- Beliefs about the medicine, or medicines in general – for example, that medicines are unnatural, harmful, addictive, or that their effects wear off over time.

NPC Plus (2007) suggests that although practical and logistical difficulties may play a part in unintentional non-compliance with medication, most non-compliance is intentional and based on a conscious decision. This includes people's beliefs about their medications, how the medicines should be used and how medicine taking fits within their daily lives. Furthermore these beliefs are shaped by a number of factors including culture, education, social circumstances, fears and anxiety, and experience of family and friends. They may misunderstand the nature of their illness and/or treatment or be unsure whether the benefits of taking the treatment outweigh the risks (NPC Plus 2007).

PAUSE FOR REFLECTION

1 If you have ever been prescribed medication did you take it exactly as prescribed, and were potential side effects explained to you and/or the potential consequences of not taking the medication as prescribed?
2 What reasons have patients given you for not wishing to take their medication? How did you deal with the situation: were you didactic or supportive in achieving mutual agreement?

In order to achieve successful concordance NPC Plus has developed a competency framework which includes eight competencies grouped into three key areas, outlined below:

- Building a partnership: patients have enough knowledge to participate as partners and health professionals are prepared for partnership.
- Managing a shared consultation: prescribing consultations involve patients as partners.
- Sharing a decision: patients are supported in taking medicines.

Development of competencies through a competency framework helps individuals improve their performance and do their jobs more effectively. The NPC Plus competency framework, accessible from the report, *A Competency Framework for Shared Decision-making with Patients: Achieving Concordance for Taking Medicines* and the website (http://www.keele.ac.uk/schools/pharm/npcplus/prescribing/Concordance.htm) may be used as a starting point for discussion of competencies either by individuals or as a group learning approach. It can help individuals and organisations identify the skills they require, including training and development needs, and inform the commissioning, development and provision of educational training programmes (NPC Plus 2007).

PAUSE FOR REFLECTION

1 Have you ever used a competency framework, either individually or as a team?
2 Using the NPC competency framework, review your learning needs related to developing concordance.

In addition to the competency framework, the Medicines Partnership Programme has produced a number of publications relating to a range of areas from medication review to project evaluation, including *Room for Review*, which focuses on medication review in primary care with a specific focus on the needs of older people and people with LTCs. These may be accessed at: http://www.keele.ac.uk/schools/pharm/npcplus/medpartpubs.htm.

CONCLUSION

Although Part Two of this chapter has concentrated mainly on initiatives relating to medicines management in England, it is appreciated that there are many innovative and effective schemes being carried out in other parts of the UK (Wales, Scotland and Northern Ireland) as well as further afield. Wales, for example, has an All Wales Medicine Strategy Group to provide advice on strategic medicines management and prescribing. However, it was felt that the

NPC programmes when summarised gave a clear overview of the types of initiatives that can support both effective medicines management and support and develop patient concordance. It would be remiss to conclude Part Two without mentioning the importance of the impact of independent non-medical prescribing by nurses and allied health professionals on medicines management as a whole. Within the UK suitably qualified nurses and pharmacists following completion of an independent prescribing programme can now legally prescribe any licensed medicine for any medical condition, within their own competencies (although there are differences in implementation in Wales, Scotland and Northern Ireland). Supplementary prescribing has been introduced for a range of other allied health professionals (physiotherapists, chiropodists/podiatrists and radiographers) to enable them to prescribe certain medicines within an agreed clinical management plan. Nurse prescribing is also established in other countries such as the USA, Australia and New Zealand; nurses from these countries should access their regulatory bodies for further information. Without doubt the introduction and extension of non-medical prescribing has had and will continue to have a huge impact on the quality of services available to people with LTCs.

KEY POINTS

- Medicines management is essential for delivery of effective health care.
- All health care professionals can play a part in delivering effective medicines management.
- Developing concordance between people with LTCs and health care professionals is essential; decision making regarding treatment options should be shared between the person with the LTC, his or her family and carer as appropriate, and the health care professional.
- Many innovative schemes have been developed to promote effective medicines management, and these should be shared and implemented among all relevant health care professionals.

FURTHER AREAS TO CONSIDER

- Think about what methods you use to develop shared decision making.
- How do you share good practice?
- Are you reluctant to adopt effective schemes developed by others in case you are seen as 'copying'? Remember: good practice is about sharing innovation to improve patient care, not keeping it to yourself!

CHAPTER 11

CONCLUSION

The overall aim of this book has been to supply a practical and useful guide to health care professionals, specifically nurses, both pre-registration and those embarking on practice nursing/community nursing careers, on the wide-ranging aspects of implementing and providing care packages and promoting self-management advice for people with long-term conditions (LTCs). This has included an overview of guiding policy, not everyone's favourite topic, but a necessary and important one to inform the reader of what is happening regarding support, care and treatment of people with long-term conditions. What is clear is that LTCs are not going away. With an increasing elderly population LTCs are set to increase, and this has clearly been identified by health and policy leaders worldwide. By the time this book is published, it is likely that more policies will have been developed, but as may be seen when reading through the pages, many of today's existing policies are not new but have just been adapted for different countries. Although innovation is always welcome we must also be careful that in developing new methods we do not throw away existing methods that work, and work well. As I mentioned in Chapter 10, we should not be afraid to both share our own good practice and adopt practices developed by others that have been shown to be successful.

My own interest in LTCs has without doubt been influenced by personal experience; diabetes looms large in my family and I am sure that most of you reading this text have had your own lives touched in one way or another by the burden of chronic disease. Prior to moving into education I had a long career in practice nursing and always felt that managing LTCs was one area where you could really make a difference. The people for whom I cared were a source of inspiration, and I continue to base my teaching on the lessons I learned from them. Avoid being judgemental and remember that no one can truly know how they would behave in a given situation. Appreciate social and cultural influences on people's lives and always treat people as individuals. If you take one message from this book I hope it is that of shared decision making and concordance, and appreciating that those who live with an LTC will have far more knowledge about its impact on their life than any health care professional can have. However, it is up to you to share your knowledge with your patients/clients and provide them with the appropriate information with which to make their own decisions. Hopefully the chapter on evidence-based practice will have improved your ability to access knowledge backed by up-to-date evidence and ensure that your practice is not based on 'unsubstantiated certainty'. This book has been about sharing knowledge, and would not have been written without utilising the excellent sources of information included in the extensive reference list. Hopefully you are now aware of sources you can add to your 'favourites' list.

Finally, remember that you are not alone; in health care we work as part of a team. Respect the knowledge of others, including your patients, their families and carers, and above all respect their wishes. The decision regarding their care is ultimately theirs and theirs alone; we can but advise and support them in the decisions they make.

REFERENCES

Acheson P. (1998) *Independent Inquiry into Inequalities in Health, The Acheson Report.* London: The Stationery Office.

Amrhein P.C., Miller W.R., Yahne C.E., Palmer M., Fulcher L. (2003) Client commitment language during motivational interviewing predicts drug use outcomes. *Journal of Consulting and Clinical Psychology* 71: 862–78.

Arthritis Australia (2008) *What is Arthritis?* accessed June 2008 from: http://arthritis australia.com.au/What%20Is%20Arthritis.

Arthritis Care (2008) *Ways to Self-manage* accessed June 2008 from: http://www.arthritis care.org.uk/LivingwithArthritis/Self-management/Waystoself-manage.

Asthma UK Cymru (2008) *A Quarter of a Million Voices . . . and Counting* accessed July 2008 from: http://www.asthma.org.uk/news_media/news/a_quarter_feel_hopel.html.

Audit Commission (1999) *First Assessment: A Review of District Nursing Services in England and Wales.* London: Audit Commission.

Australian Government Department of Health and Ageing (2006) *Factbook 2006* accessed 2008 from: http://www.health.gov.au/internet/wcms/publishing.nsf/Content/Factbook2006-1~factbook2006-ch5-introduction~chapter5-sect-9.

Australian Government Department of Health and Ageing (2007) *Sharing Health Care Initiative* accessed 2008 from: http://www.health.gov.au/internet/main/Publishing.nsf/Content/chronicdisease-sharing.htm.

Australian Institute of Health and Welfare (AIHW) (2005) *Chronic Diseases* accessed 2008 from: http://www.aihw.gov.au/cdarf/data_pages/oecd/index.cfm.

Bandura A.E. (1995) *Self-efficacy in Changing Societies.* New York: Cambridge University Press.

Barasi M. (2003) *Human Nutrition: A Health Perspective* (2nd edn). London: Arnold Publishers.

Barlow J., Wright C., Sheasby J., Turner A., Hainsworth J. (2002) Self-management approaches for people with chronic conditions: a review. *Patient Education Counselling* 4 (48): 177–87.

Bem D.J. (1972) Self-perception theory. In L. Berkowitz (ed.) *Advances in Experimental Social Psychology.* New York: Academic Press.

Bennett J., Robinson A. (2005) District nursing: evolution or extinction. *Journal of Community Nursing* 19 (4): 26–8.

Bent N., Tennant A., Swift T., Posnett J., Scuffham P. and A.M.P., Chamberlain M.A. (2000) Team approach versus ad-hoc health services for young people with physical disabilities: a retrospective cohort study. *Lancet* 360: 1280–6.

Bernabei E., Landi F., Gamgassi G. (1998) Randomised trial of impact model of integrated care and case management for older people living in the community. *British Medical Journal* 2 (316): 1348–51.

Bidwell S. (2004) Finding the evidence: resources and skills for locating information on clinical effectiveness. *Singapore Medical Journal* 45 (12): 567–72.

Blaxter M. (1990) *Health and Lifestyles*. London: Routledge.

BMJ Clinical Evidence (2008) *BMJ Clinical Evidence* accessed July 2008 from: http://clinicalevidence.bmj.com/ceweb/index.jsp.

Boaden R., Dusheiko M., Gravelle H., Parker S., Pickard S., Roland M., Sargent P., Sheaff R. (2006) *Evaluation of Evercare: Final Report*. University of Manchester: National Primary Care Research and Development Centre accessed June 2008 from: http://www.npcrdc.ac.uk/Publications/evercare_final_report.pdf.

Bodenheimer T., Lorig K., Holman H., Grumbach K. (2002) Patient self-management of chronic disease in primary care. *Journal of American Medical Association* 288: 2469–75.

Brehm J.W. (1966) *A Theory of Psychological Reactance*. New York: Academic Press.

British Dietetic Association (BDA) (1997) Position Paper. Obesity Treatment: Future Directions for the Contribution of Dieticians. London: BDA.

British Heart Foundation (2008) *Cardiovascular Disease* accessed July 2008 from: http://www.bhf.org.uk/living_with_heart_conditions/understanding_heart_conditions/types_of_heart_conditions/coronary_heart_disease.aspx.

British Lung Foundation (2007) *COPD* accessed July 2008 from: http://www.lunguk.org/you-and-your-lungs/conditions-and-diseases/copd.htm.

British Medical Association (BMA)/NHS Confederation (2003) *Investing in General Practice: The GMS Contract*. London: BMA.

British Medical Association (BMA) (2004) *Diabetes Mellitus: An Update for Healthcare Professionals*. London: BMA.

British Medical Journal (BMJ) (2000) Patients as partners in managing chronic disease. *British Medical Journal* 320: 526–7.

British Thoracic Society/SIGN (2008) *British Guideline on the Management of Asthma* accessed July 2008 from: http://www.brit-thoracic.org.uk/ClinicalInformation/Asthma/AsthmaGuidelines/tabid/83/Default.aspx.

Burke B., Arkowitz H., Menchola M. (2003) The efficacy of motivational interviewing: a meta-analysis of controlled clinical trials. *Journal of Consulting and Clinical Psychology* 71: 843–61.

Centres for Disease Control and Prevention (CDCP) (2007) *Chronic Disease Prevention* accessed 2008 from: http://www.cdc.gov/nccdphp/index.htm.

Centre for Economic Policy Research (2008) *Does Unemployment Damage your Health?* London: CEPR.

Centre for Research and Dissemination (CRD) (2005) *About CRD Databases* accessed July 2008 from: http://www.crd.york.ac.uk/crdweb/html/help.htm.

Chowdhury T. (2003) Preventing diabetes in south Asians: too little action and too late. *British Medical Journal* 327 (7423): 1059–60.

Clinical Knowledge Summaries (CKS) (2005) *Rheumatoid Arthritis* accessed July 2008 from: http://www.prodigy.nhs.uk/rheumatoid_arthritis/making_a_diagnosis/diagnosis/clinical_features#-188990.

Clinical Knowledge Summaries (CKS) (2006a) *Heart Failure* accessed July 2008 from: http://cks.library.nhs.uk/heart_failure#-217145.

Clinical Knowledge Summaries (CKS) (2006b) *Epilepsy* accessed July 2008 from: http://cks.library.nhs.uk/epilepsy#-238865.

Clinical Knowledge Summaries (CKS) (2006c) *Osteoporosis* accessed July 2008 from: http://www.prodigy.nhs.uk/osteoporosis_treatment#-221285.

Clinical Knowledge Summaries (CKS) (2007a) *Asthma* accessed July 2008 from: http://www.cks.library.nhs.uk/asthma#-297066.

Clinical Knowledge Summaries (CKS) (2007b) *Angina* accessed August 2008 from: http://www.cks.library.nhs.uk/angina#-238810.

Clinical Knowledge Summaries (CKS) (2008a) *Eczema* accessed July 2008 from: http://cks.library.nhs.uk/eczema_atopic.

Clinical Knowledge Summaries (CKS) (2008b) *Osteoarthritis* accessed August 2008 from: http://www.cks.library.nhs.uk/osteoarthritis/management/quick_answers/scenario_ost eoarthritis/clinical_summary_all_joints_management/drug_treatments#-324225.

Cochrane Collaboration, The (2008) *Archie Cochrane: The Name Behind the Cochrane Collaboration* accessed July 2008 from: http://www.cochrane.org/docs/archieco. htm.

Corbin S., Rosen R. (2005) *Self-management for Long-term Conditions*. London: King's Fund.

Craig P. (2002) The development of public health nursing. In S. Cowley, *Public Health in Policy and Practice: A Sourcebook for Health Visitors and Community Nurses*. London: Bailliere Tindall.

Cullum N. (2000) Users' guide to the nursing literature: an introduction. *Evidence Based Nursing* 3 (3): 71–2.

Dahlgren G., Whitehead M. (1991) *Policies and Strategies to Promote Social Equity in Health*. Stockholm: Institute for Future Studies.

Department for Environment, Food and Rural Affairs (2008) *Departmental Report*. London: DEFRA Cm 7399.

Department of Health (DoH) (1990) *General Medical Services Council: New GP Contract*. London: HMSO.

Department of Health (DoH) (1991) *Research for Health: A Research and Development Strategy for the NHS*. London: HMSO.

Department of Health (DoH) (1992) *The Health of the Nation*. London: HMSO.

Department of Health (DoH) (1997) *The New NHS: Modern, Dependable*. London: The Stationery Office.

Department of Health (DoH) (1998) *A First Class Service: Quality in the New NHS*. London: HMSO.

Department of Health (DoH) (1999) *Saving Lives: Our Healthier Nation*. London: Department of Health.

Department of Health (DoH) (2000a) *National Service Framework for Coronary Heart Disease*. London: HMSO.

Department of Health (DoH) (2000b) *The NHS Plan: A Plan for Investment, a Plan for Reform*. London: HMSO.

Department of Health (DoH) (2000c) *Pharmacy in the Future*. London: HMSO.

Department of Health (DoH) (2001) *The Expert Patient: A New Approach to Chronic Disease Management for the 21st Century*. London: Department of Health Publications.

Department of Health (DoH) (2002) *National Service Framework for Diabetes*. London: Department of Health Publications.

Department of Health (DoH) (2004a) *Chronic Disease Management*. London: Department of Health Publications.

Department of Health (DoH) (2004b) *The NHS Improvement Plan: Putting People at the Heart of Public Services*. London: Department of Health Publications.

Department of Health (DoH) (2005a) *Supporting People with Long Term Conditions. Liberating the Talents of Nurses who Care for People with Long Term Conditions.* London: Department of Health Publications.

Department of Health (DoH) (2005b) *DH MORI Survey: Public Attitudes to Self Care Baseline Survey.* London: Department of Health Publications.

Department of Health (DoH) (2005c) *Supporting People with Long Term Conditions. An NHS Social Care Model to Support Local Innovation and Integration.* London: Department of Health Publications.

Department of Health (DoH) (2005d) *National Service Framework for Long Term Conditions* accessed July 2008 from: http://www.dh.gov.uk/en/Publicationsandstatistics /Publications/PublicationsPolicyAndGuidance/DH_4105361.

Department of Health (DoH) (2005e) *Health Survey of England 2005.* London: Department of Health Publications.

Department of Health (DoH) (2006a) *Our Health, Our Care, Our Say: A New Direction for Community Services.* London: Department of Health Publications.

Department of Health (DoH) (2006b) *The Expert Patients Programme* accessed June 2008 from: http://www.dh.gov.uk/en/Aboutus/MinistersandDepartmentLeaders/Chief MedicalOfficer/ProgressOnPolicy/ProgressBrowsableDocument/DH_4102757.

Department of Health (DoH) (2007) *Long Term Conditions* accessed 2008 from: http://www.dh.gov.uk/en/Policyandguidance/Healthandsocialcaretopics/Longterm conditions/index.htm.

Department of Health (DoH) (2008a) *National Service Frameworks (NSFs)* accessed 2008 from: http://www.dh.gov.uk/en/ArchivedSections/Healthandsocialcaretopics/ DH_4070951.

Department of Health (DoH) (2008b) *Raising the Profile of Long Term Conditions Care: A Compendium of Information.* London: Department of Health Publications.

Department of Health, Social Services and Public Safety (2005) *A Healthier Future: A Twenty Year Vision for Health and Well-being in Northern Ireland* accessed 2008 from http://www.dhsspsni.gov.uk/healthyfuture-section2.pdf.

Diabetes UK (2006) *Long Term Complications* accessed June 2008 from: http://www. diabetes.org.uk/Guide-to-diabetes/Complications/Long_term_complications/.

Donnelly L. (2008) *Don't Treat the Old and Unhealthy, say Doctors* accessed July 2008 from: http://www. telegraph.co.uk.

Drennan V., Goodman C. (2004) Nurse-led case management for older people with long-term conditions. *British Journal of Community Nursing* 9 (12): 527–33.

Dunn C., Deroo L., Rivara F. (2001) The use of brief interventions adapted from motivational interviewing across behavioral domains: a systematic review. *Addiction* 96: 1725–42.

EdRen (Renal Unit of the Royal Infirmary of Edinburgh) (2006) *End Stage Renal Failure and its Treatment* accessed July 2008 from: http://renux.dmed.ed.ac.uk/EdREN/ EdRenINFObits/Dialysis_ESRFLong.html.

Effing T.W., Monninkhof E.M., van der Valk P.D.L.P.M., Zielhuis G.A., van Herwaarden C.L.A., Partridge M.R., Walters E.H., van der Palen J. (2007) Self-management education for patients with chronic obstructive pulmonary disease. *Cochrane Database of Systematic Reviews* 4.

Elder A., Holmes J. (2002) *Mental Health in Primary Care.* New York: Oxford University Press.

Epilepsy Action (2008) *About Take Control* accessed August 2008 from: http://www. takecontroluk.org/asp/template_abouttakecontrol.asp?id=30&sm=.

Expert Patients Programme Wales (2008) accessed June 2008 from: http://www.wales. nhs.uk/sites3/home.cfm?orgid=537.

Fahey T., Schroeder K., Ebrahim S. (2006) Interventions used to improve control of blood pressure in patients with hypertension. *Cochrane Database of Systematic Reviews* 2.

Festinger L. (1957) *A Theory of Cognitive Dissonance.* Stanford, CA: Stanford University Press.

Flemming K. (1998) Asking answerable questions. *Evidence Based Nursing* 1(2): 36–7.

Foster G., Taylor S.J.C., Eldridge S.E., Ramsay J., Griffiths C.J. (2007) Self-management education programmes by lay leaders for people with chronic conditions. *Cochrane Database of Systematic Reviews* 4.

Friedson E. (1970) *Profession of Medicine: A Study of the Sociology of Applied Knowledge.* New York: Harper & Row.

Gagnon L. (1999) Quantitative measurement of caring. *Journal of Advanced Nursing* 36: 390–5.

Government Equalities Office (2008) *Gender Pay Gap* accessed July 2008 from: http://www.equalities.gov.uk/women_work/pay.htm.

Greenhalgh T. (2001) *How to Read a Paper: The Basics of Evidence Based Medicine* (2nd edn). London: BMJ.

Griffin S. (2001) The management of diabetes: moving beyond registration, recall, and regular review. *British Medical Journal* 323: 970–5.

Griffin S., Kinmonth A.L. (2000) Systems for routine surveillance for people with diabetes mellitus. *Cochrane Database of Systematic Reviews* 2.

Halpin D. (2008) *COPD: Journal of Chronic Obstructive Pulmonary Disease* 5 (3): 187–200 accessed July 2008 from: http://www.informaworld.com/smpp/section? content=a793961775&fulltext=713240928.

Handley M., MacGregor K., Schillinger D., Sharifi C., Wong S., Bodenheimer T. (2006) Using action plans to help primary care patients adopt healthy behaviors: a descriptive study. *The Journal of the American Board of Family Medicine* 19: 224–31.

Hettema J., Steele J., Miller W.R. (2005) Motivational interviewing. *Annual Review of Clinical Psychology* 1: 91–111.

Hill-Briggs F. and Gemmell L. (2007) Problem solving in diabetes self-management and control. *The Diabetes Educator* 33 (6): 1032–50.

Holman H., Lorig K. (2000) Patients as partners in managing chronic disease. *British Medical Journal* 320 (7234): 526–7.

Hutt R., Rosen R., McCauley J. (2004) *Case-managing Long-term Conditions.* London: King's Fund.

Illich I. (1976) *Limits to Medicine.* London: Marion Boyars.

Improvement Foundation (2008) *Long-term Conditions* accessed July 2008 from: http://www.improvementfoundation.org/theme/long-term-conditions.

International Diabetes Federation (IDF) (2007) *Diabetes Facts and Figures* accessed June 2008 from: http://www.idf.org/home/index.cfm?node=6.

Jackson G., Yano E., Edelman, D., Krein S.L., Ibrahim M.A., Carey T.S., Lee S.D., Hartmann K.E., Dudley T.K., Weinberger M. (2005) Veterans affairs primary care organizational characteristics associated with better diabetic control. *American Journal of Managed Care* 11: 225–37.

Joanna Briggs Institute (2008) *The JBI Approach to Evidence-based Practice* accessed July 2008 from: http://www.joannabriggs.edu.au/about/system_review.php.

Jung R. (1997) Obesity as a disease. *British Medical Bulletin* 53(2): 307–21.

Keller V., White M. (1997) Choices and changes: a new model for influencing patient health behavior. *Journal of Clinical Outcomes Management* 4: 33–6.

Knight K., McGowan L., Dickens C., Bundy C. (2006) A systematic review of motivational interviewing in physical health care settings. *British Journal of Health Psychology* 11: 319–32.

Lane C., Huws-Thomas M., Hood K., Rollnick S., Edwards K., Robling M. (2005)

Measuring adaptations of motivational interviewing: the development and validation of the Behavior Change Counseling Index. *Patient Education and Counselling* 56: 166–73.

Litaker D., Moin L.C. (2003) Physician–nurse practitioner teams in chronic disease management: the impact on cost, clinical effectiveness and patients' reception of care. *Journal of Inter-professional Care* 17 (3): 221–37.

Lorig K.R., Sobel D.S., Stewart A.L., Brown Jr B.W., Ritter P.L., González V.M., Laurent D.D., Holman H.R. (1999) Evidence suggesting that a chronic disease self-management program can improve health status while reducing utilization and costs: a randomized trial. *Medical Care* 37 (1): 5–14.

Lyons C., Nixon D., Coren A. (2006) *Long-term Conditions and Depression.* London: Care Services Improvement Partnership (CSIP).

McAlister F., Stewart S., Ferrua S., McMurray J. (2004) Multidisciplinary strategies for the management of heart failure patients at high risk for admission. *Journal of the American College of Cardiology* 44: 810–19.

McKenzie K. (2003) Racism and health. *British Medical Journal* 326: 65–6.

Madson M.B., Campbell T.C., Barrett D.E., Brondino M.J., Melchert T.P. (2005) Development of the Motivational Interviewing Supervision and Training Scale. *Psychology of Addictive Behaviors* 19: 303–10.

Mayor S. (2007) The impact of depression on life for people with Parkinson's disease. *British Journal of Neuroscience Nursing* 3 (11): 512–14.

Miller W., Rollnick S. (2002) *Motivational Interviewing: Preparing People for Change.* New York: Guilford Press.

Miller W.R., Benefield R.G., Tonigan J.S. (1993) Enhancing motivation for change in problem drinking: a controlled comparison of two therapist styles. *Journal of Consulting and Clinical Psychology* 61: 455–61.

Ministry of Health New Zealand (2008) *Long-term Conditions Programme* accessed June 2008 from: http://www.moh.govt.nz/longtermconditions.

Moyers T., Martin T., Manuel J., Hendrickson S., Miller W. (2005) Assessing competence in the use of motivational interviewing. *Journal of Substance Abuse Treatment* 28: 19–26.

Najavitis L.M., Crits-Christoph P. (2000) Clinicians' impact on the quality of substance use disorder treatment. *Substance Use and Misuse* 35: 2161–90.

National Centre for Chronic Disease Prevention and Health Promotion (2008) *Arthritis* accessed June 2008 from: http://www.cdc.gov/arthritis/.

National Collaborating Centre for Chronic Conditions (2006) *Parkinson's: National Clinical Guidelines for Care and Management in Adults.* London: Royal College of Physicians.

National Collaborating Centre for Chronic Conditions (2008) *Osteoarthritis: National Clinical Guidelines for Care and Management in Adults.* London: Royal College of Physicians.

National Health Priority Action Council (NHPAC) (2006) *National Chronic Disease Strategy.* Canberra: Australian Government Department of Health and Ageing.

National Institute of Health and Clinical Excellence (NICE) (2002) *Principles for Best Practice in Clinical Audit.* Oxford: Radcliffe.

National Institute of Health and Clinical Excellence (NICE) (2003) *Chronic Heart Failure* accessed July 2008 from: http://www.nice.org.uk/Guidance/CG5.

National Institute of Health and Clinical Excellence (NICE) (2004a) *Depression* accessed July 2008 from: http://www.nice.org.uk/Guidance/CG23/Guidance/pdf/English.

National Institute of Health and Clinical Excellence (NICE) (2004b) *Type 1 Diabetes: Diagnosis and Management of Type 1 Diabetes in Adults* accessed June 2008 from: http://www.nice.org.uk/Guidance/CG15/QuickRefGuide/pdf/English.

National Institute of Health and Clinical Excellence (NICE) (2004c) *Epilepsy in Children and Adults* accessed July 2008 from: http://www.nice.org.uk/Guidance/CG20/ NiceGuidance/pdf/English.

National Institute of Health and Clinical Excellence (NICE) (2004d) *Management of Chronic Obstructive Pulmonary Disease in Adults in Primary and Secondary Care* accessed July 2008 from: http://www.nice.org.uk/Guidance/CG12.

National Institute of Health and Clinical Excellence (NICE) (2006a) *Hypertension: Management of Hypertension in Adults in Primary Care* accessed July 2008 from: http://www.nice.org.uk/CG034.

National Institute for Health and Clinical Excellence (NICE) (2006b) *Guideline 43: Obesity: The Prevention, Identification, Assessment and Management of Overweight and Obesity in Adults and Children* accessed July 2008 from: http://www.nice.org.uk/ guidance/index.jsp?action=byID&o=11000.

National Institute of Health and Clinical Excellence (NICE) (2007) *Clinical Guidelines* accessed March 2008 from: http://www.nice.org.uk/guidance/index.jsp?action= byTopic.

National Institute of Health and Clinical Excellence (NICE) (2008) *Diabetes – Type 2* accessed July 2008 from: http://www.nice.org.uk/Guidance/CG66.

National Obesity Forum (2008) *Guidelines on Management of Adult Obesity and Overweight in Primary Care* accessed July 2008 from www.nationalobesityforum. org.uk.

National Prescribing Centre (NPC) (2002) Medicines management services – why are they so important? *MeReC Bulletin* 12(6): 21–4.

National Prescribing Centre (NPC) (2005) *MMS Collaborative Wave 3 Review Final Report*. Liverpool: NPC.

National Prescribing Centre (NPC) (2007) *Community Pharmacy Framework Collaborative (CPFC) Final Report*. Liverpool: NPC.

National Society for Epilepsy (2007) *Information on Epilepsy: What is Epilepsy?* accessed July 2008 from: http://www.epilepsynse.org.uk/PAGES/info/leaflets/explaini.cfm.

Nettleton S. (2006) *The Sociology of Health and Illness* (2nd edn). Cambridge: Polity Press.

NHS Executive (1999) Asking the question: finding the evidence. *Evidence-based Health Care*. Unit 2. Luton: CASP/HCLU.

NHS Institute for Innovation and Improvement (2006) *Improving Care for People with Long Term Conditions* accessed 2008 from: http://www.hsmc.bham.ac.uk/news/ ReviewIntFrameworks-ltc.pdf.

Northern Ireland Executive (2008) *Press Release – Major £46 Million Investment in Chronic Conditions* accessed 2008 from: http://www.northernireland.gov.uk/news/ news-dhssps/news-dhssps-220108-major-46million-investment.htm.

NPC Plus (2007) *A Competency Framework for Shared Decision-making with Patients: Achieving Concordance for Taking Medicines*. Liverpool: NPC.

Oakley A. (1993) *Essays on Women, Medicine and Health*. Edinburgh: Edinburgh University Press.

Office for National Statistics (ONS) (2002) *Mental Health of Carers*. London: Stationery Office

Office for National Statistics (ONS) (2004) *Geographic Inequalities in Life Expectancy Persist across the United Kingdom*. London: ONS.

Office for National Statistics (ONS) (2005) *National Statistics Online* accessed July 2008 from: http://www.statistics.gov.uk/.

Olivarius N. de F., Beck-Nielsen H., Andreasen A.H., Horder M., Pedersen P.A. (2001) Randomised controlled trial of structured personal care of type 2 diabetes mellitus. *British Medical Journal* 323: 970–5.

Parsons T. (1951) *The Social System*. Glencoe, IL: Free Press.

Patient UK (2006) *Diabetic Ketoacidosis* accessed July 2008 from: http://www.patient.co.uk/showdoc/40001335/.

Patient UK (2008) *Hyperosmolar Hyperglycaemic Non-ketotic Coma (HONK)* accessed July 2008 from: http://www.patient.co.uk/showdoc/40025333/.

Patterson E., Muenchenberger H., Kendall E. (2007) The role of practice nurses in co-ordinated care of people with chronic and complex conditions. *Australian Health Review* 31 (2): 231–8.

Powell H., Gibson P.G. (2002) Options for self-management education for adults with asthma. *Cochrane Database of Systematic Reviews* 3.

Prochaska J.O., DiClemente C.C. (1983) Stages and processes of self-change of smoking: toward an integrative model of change. *Journal of Consulting and Clinical Psychology* 51: 390–5.

Psoriasis Association, The (2008) *What is Psoriasis?* accessed July 2008 from: http://www.psoriasis-association.org.uk/what-is.html.

RCGP (2004) *RCGP Information Sheet No. 19: Practice Nurses* accessed August 2007 from: http://www.rcgp.org.uk/pdf/ISS_INFO_19_AUG%2004.pdf.

Redhead K. (2003) Perspectives from a developed nation. *Epilepsia* 44 (Suppl 1): 51–4.

Rees J., O'Boyle C., MacDonagh R. (2001) Quality of life: impact of chronic illness on the partner. *Journal of the Royal Society of Medicine* 94(11): 563–6.

Rees S., Williams A. (2008) Promoting and supporting self-care management for adults living in the community with physical chronic illness: the effectiveness and meaningfulness of the patient–practitioner encounter. *Joanna Briggs Institute Database of Systematic Reviews*.

Renal Association (2007) *Stages of CKD (Chronic Kidney Disease)* accessed July 2008 from: http://www.renal.org/eGFR/ckdstages.html.

Renders C.M., Valk G.D., Griffin S.J., Wagner E.H., Eijk Van J.T., Assendelft W.J. (2001) Interventions to improve the management of diabetes mellitus in primary care, outpatient and community settings. *Cochrane Database of Systematic Reviews* 2.

Rethink (2006) *Self-management* accessed June 2008 from: http://www.rethink.org/living_with_mental_illness/recovery_and_self_management/selfmanagement/index.html.

Riemsma R.P., Kirwan J.R., Taal E., Rasker J.J. (2003) Patient education for adults with rheumatoid arthritis. *Cochrane Database of Systematic Reviews* 2.

Robb G., Seddon M. (2006) Quality improvement in New Zealand healthcare. Part 6: Keeping the patient front and centre to improve healthcare quality. *Journal of the New Zealand Medical Association* 119 (1242), http://www.nzma.org.nz/journal/119-1242/2174/.

Rollnick S., Mason P., Butler C. (1999) *Health Behaviour Change: A Guide for Practitioners*. Edinburgh: Harcourt Brace.

Rollnick S., Miller W., Butler C. (2007) *Motivational Interviewing in Healthcare*. New York: Guilford Press.

Royal Pharmaceutical Society of Great Britain and the British Medical Association (BMA) (2000) *Teamworking in Primary Healthcare – Final Report*. London: Royal Pharmaceutical Society of Great Britain and the British Medical Association.

Rubak S., Sandboek A., Lauritzen T., Christensen B. (2005) Motivational interviewing: a systematic review and meta-analysis. *British Journal of General Practice* 55: 305–12.

Sackett D.L., Rosenberg W.M., Muir Gray J.A., Haynes R.B., Richardson W.S. (1996) Evidence-based medicine: what it is and what it isn't. *British Medical Journal* 312: 71–2.

Sackett D.L., Straus S.E., Richardson W.S., Rosenberg W., Haynes R.B. (2000) *Evidence Based Medicine: How to Practice and Teach EBM* (2nd edn). Edinburgh: Churchill-Livingstone.

Scottish Government (2007a) *Characteristics of Adults in Scotland with Long Term Conditions: An Analysis of Scottish Household and Scottish Health Surveys* accessed 2008 from: http://www.scotland.gov.uk/Publications/2007/10/29093311/0.

Scottish Government (2007b) *Living Well with Long Term Conditions* accessed 2008 from: http://www.scotland.gov.uk/Publications/2007/12/24104752/10.

Scottish Government (2008) *Better Health Better Care Action Plan: What it Means for You.* Edinburgh: Scottish Government.

Scottish Intercollegiate Guidelines Network (SIGN) (2004) *Management of Osteoporosis* accessed August 2008 from: http://www.sign.ac.uk/guidelines/fulltext/71/index.html

Scottish Intercollegiate Guidelines Network (SIGN) (2006) *Diagnosis and Management of Peripheral Arterial Disease* accessed July 2008 from: www.sign.ac.uk/pdf/sign89.pdf.

Scottish Intercollegiate Guidelines Network (SIGN) (2008) *Diagnosis and Management of Chronic Kidney Disease* accessed July 2008 from: http://www.renal.org/pages/media/Guidelines/sign103.pdf.

Sheehy C., Murphy E., Barry M. (2006) Depression in rheumatoid arthritis: underscoring the problem. *Rheumatology* 45: 1325–7.

Stanford University School of Medicine Patient Education Research Centre (2008) *Chronic Disease Self-management Program* accessed June 2008 from: http://patient education.stanford.edu/programs/cdsmp.html.

Stokes T., Shaw E.J., Camosso-Stefinovic J., Baker R., Baker G.A., Jacoby A. (2007) Self-management education for children with epilepsy. *Cochrane Database of Systematic Reviews* 2.

Stroke Association, The (2008) *Common Problems* accessed July 2008 from: http://www.stroke.org.uk/information/what_is_a_stroke/common_problems.html.

Thomas B., Bishop J. (2007) *The Manual of Dietetic Practice* (4th edn). Oxford: Blackwell Publishing.

Thompson H., Ryan A. (2008) A review of the psychosocial consequences of stroke and their impact on spousal relationships. *British Journal of Neuroscience Nursing* 4(4): 177–84.

Toelle B.G., Ram F.S.F. (2004) Written individualised management plans for asthma in children and adults. *Cochrane Database of Systematic Reviews* 1.

Tudor-Hart J. (1971) The Inverse Care Law. *The Lancet*, 27 February: 405–12.

Turnock A.C., Walters E.H., Walters J.A.E., Wood-Baker R. (2005) Action plans for chronic obstructive pulmonary disease. *Cochrane Database of Systematic Reviews* 4.

UNICEF (2007) *The State of the World's Children, 2008. Child Survival.* New York: UNICEF.

van Dam H.A., van der Horst F., van den Borne B., Ryckman R., Crebolder H. (2003) Provider–patient interaction in diabetes care: effects on patient self-care outcomes: a systematic review. *Patient Education and Counselling* 51 (1): 17–28.

Vasilaki E., Hosier S., Cox W. (2006) The efficacy of motivational interviewing as a brief intervention for excessive drinking: a meta-analytic review. *Alcohol and Alcoholism* 41 (3): 328–35.

Wagner E.H. (1998) Chronic disease management: what will it take to improve care for chronic illness? *Effective Clinical Practice* 1: 2–4.

Wagner E.H., Austin B.T., Davis C., Hindmarsh M., Schaefer J., Bonomi A. (2001) Improving chronic illness care: translating evidence into action. *Health Affairs* 20 (6): 64–78.

Welsh Assembly Government (2001) *Improving Health in Wales: A Plan for the NHS with its Partners.* Cardiff: WAG.

Welsh Assembly Government (2005) *Designed for Life: A World Class Health Service for Wales.* Cardiff: WAG.

Welsh Assembly Government (2006a) *Chronic Disease Management* accessed 2008 from: http://wales.gov.uk/topics/health/nhswales/majorhealth/chronic_disease_management/?lang=en.

Welsh Assembly Government (2006b) *National Service Framework for Older People in Wales*. Cardiff: Welsh Assembly Government.

Welsh Assembly Government/National Public Health Service – Wales (WAG/NPHS) (2005) *A Profile of Long Term and Chronic Conditions in Wales*. Cardiff: WAG.

While A. (2007) Lessons from the Evercare evaluation. *British Journal of Community Nursing* 12(1): 46.

Williams B., Poulter N.R., Brown M.J., Davis M., McInnes G.T., Potter J.P., Sever P.S., Thom S. McG. (2004) The BHS Guidelines: Working Party Guidelines for Management of Hypertension: Report of the Fourth Working Party of the British Hypertension Society, 2004 – BHS IV. *Journal of Human Hypertension* 18: 139–85.

Wilson P.M. (2005) Long-term conditions: making sense of the current policy agenda. *British Journal of Community Nursing* 10(12): 544–52.

Wilson T., Buck D., Ham C. (2005) Rising to the challenge: will the NHS support people with long term conditions? *British Medical Journal* 330: 657–61.

World Health Organisation (1978) *The Declaration of Alma Ata. International Conference on Primary Health Care*. Alma Ata: WHO.

World Health Organisation (1986) *Ottawa Charter for Health Promotion*. Ottawa: WHO.

World Health Organisation (1991) *Community Involvement in Health Development: Challenging Health Services*. Geneva: WHO.

World Health Organisation (1998) *Obesity: Preventing and Managing the Global Epidemic*. Geneva: WHO.

World Health Organisation (2002a) *The Impact of Chronic Disease in New Zealand* accessed 2008 from: http://www.who.int/chp/chronic_disease_report/media/impact/new_zealand.pdf.

World Health Organisation (2002b) *Innovative Care for Chronic Conditions* accessed January 2008 from: http://www.who.int/diabetesactiononline/about/icccglobalreport.pdf.

World Health Organisation (2006a) *COPD: Burden* accessed July 2008 from: http://www.who.int/respiratory/copd/burden/en/index.htm.

World Health Organisation (2006b) *Definition and Diagnosis of Diabetes Mellitus and Intermediate Hyperglycaemia* accessed July 2008 from: http://www.who.int/diabetes/publications/Definition%20and%20diagnosis%20of%20diabetes_new.pdf.

World Health Organisation Regional Office for Europe (2007) *Press Release* accessed 2008 from: http://www.euro.who.int/mediacentre/PR/2006/20060908_1.

INDEX

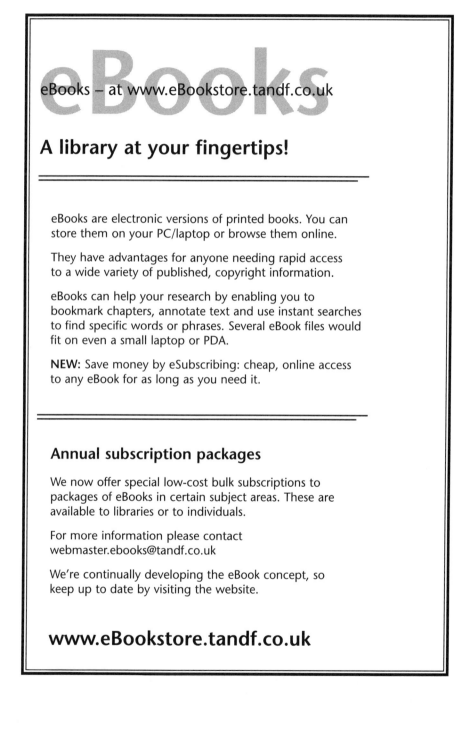

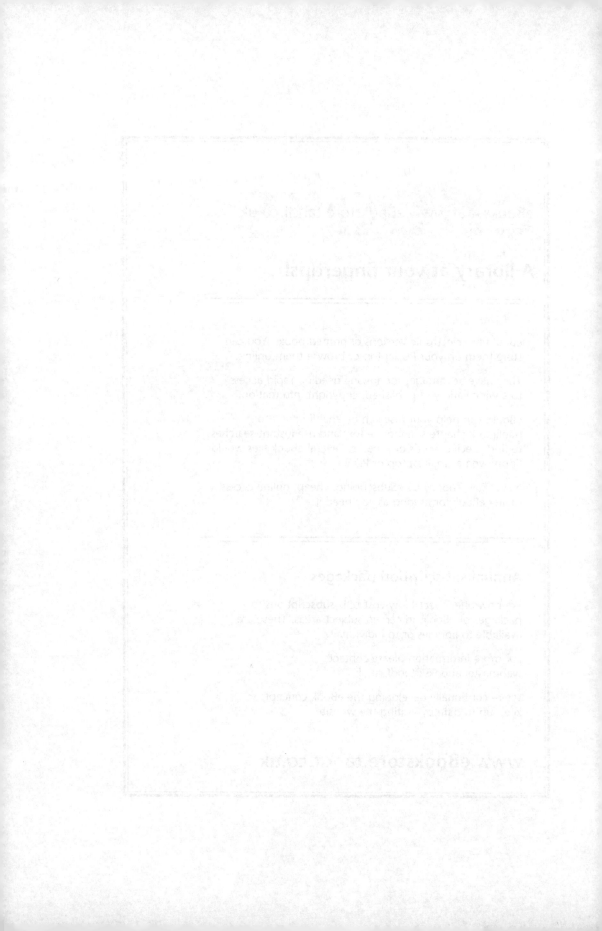